The Complete

Air Fryer Cookbook 2023

1600 Days Mouth-watering Recipes for Beginners, Quick, Less Greasy and Crispy for a Healthier Way of Cooking to Enhance Flavour

Norma S. Ibarra

CONTENTS

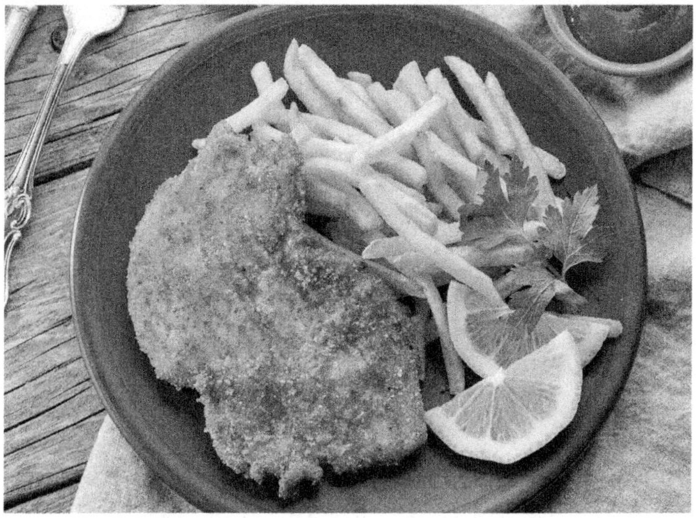

INTRODUCTION

Welcome! I'm Norma S. Ibarra, your guide on this flavor-filled journey towards a healthier lifestyle. If you know me, you know how passionately I believe in the power of good food to nourish not just our bodies, but also our souls. Well, I'm here to tell you that good food doesn't have to come at the expense of your health. And it certainly doesn't have to be complicated or time-consuming!

With this new cookbook and the magic of your air fryer, I'm going to show you how easy it is to create dishes that are as delicious as they are nutritious. The air fryer is not just a gadget; it's a transformative tool in our kitchens that has the power to change the way we cook and eat, and even the way we think about food.

Inside this cookbook, you will find a wide array of meticulously curated recipes that showcase the versatility of the air fryer. Whether it's crispy vegetables, succulent poultry, mouthwatering seafood, or delectable desserts, these dishes are designed to satisfy your cravings while keeping health in check.

From breakfast to dessert, each dish is not just a recipe; it's a celebration of fresh ingredients, bold flavors, and the joy that comes from creating and sharing good food. Along the way, you'll learn how to make the most of your air fryer with tips, tricks, and a dash of inspiration to help you make these recipes truly your own.

So, let's preheat our air fryers and roll up our sleeves. It's time to embark on a culinary adventure together, and I couldn't be more excited to guide you on this journey towards healthier, more vibrant, and most importantly, delicious cooking.

Is Air Fryer healthier?

- **Less Oil:**

Air fryers work by circulating hot air around the food to create a crispy outer layer. This process requires significantly less oil than traditional frying methods, reducing the overall fat and calorie content of the food.

- **Reduced Risk of Harmful Compounds**

Frying food at high temperatures can lead to the formation of harmful compounds, such as acrylamide, which is associated with the risk of certain diseases. Since air frying requires lower temperatures, it can potentially reduce the formation of these compounds.

- **Weight Management**

Due to the lower fat and calorie content of air-fried foods, incorporating air-fried dishes into your diet may support weight management efforts.

Preserves Nutrients

Some cooking methods can lead to a significant loss of nutrients from food. As air frying is a relatively quick method, it can help to preserve certain nutrients that are sensitive to heat.

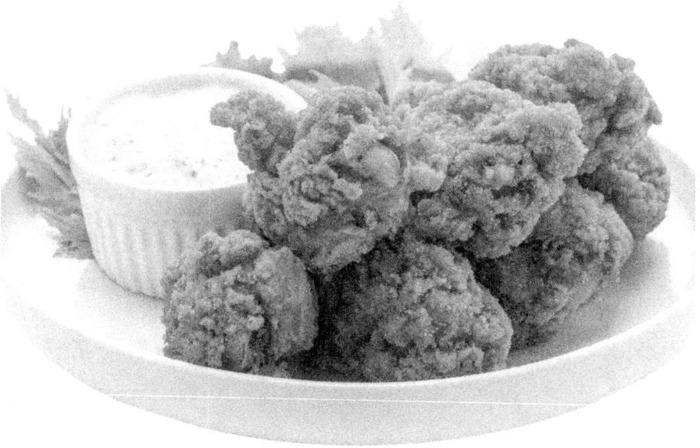

What recipes does this cookbook offer?

The "Air Fryer Diet Cookbook" features a vast collection of carefully curated, health-conscious recipes that showcase the versatility and convenience of Air Fryer.

- **Breakfast**

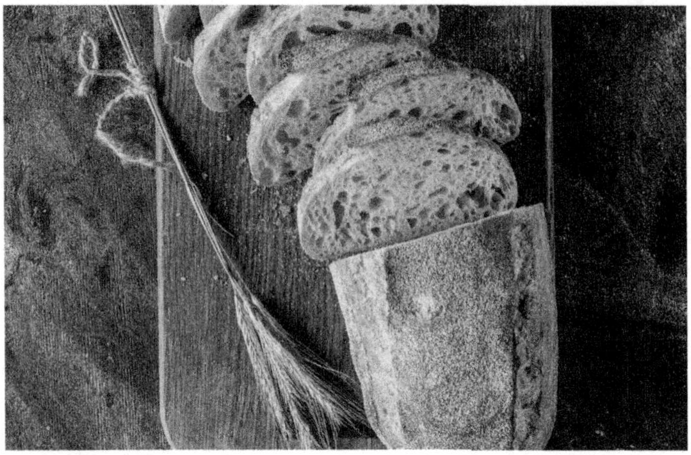

Start your day with flavorful, nutritious breakfast dishes such as French Toast Sticks, Vegetable Frittatas, or Air Fryer Granola.

- **Snacks and Appetizers**

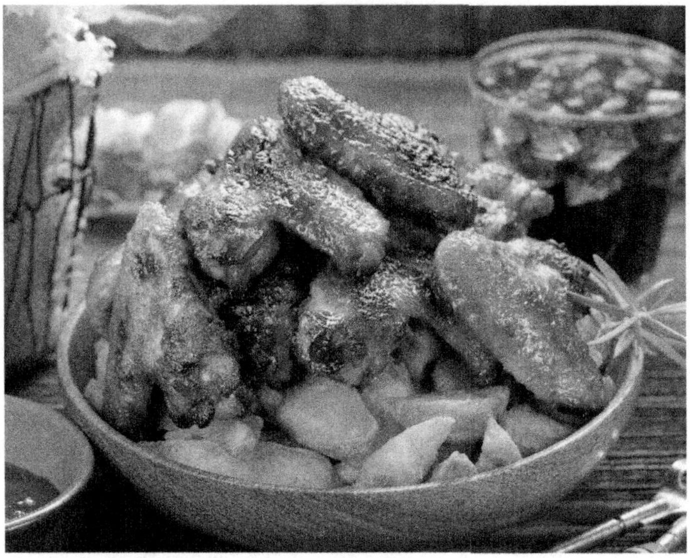

Explore a variety of bite-sized delights like Crispy Kale Chips, Spicy Chicken Wings, and Sweet Potato Fries.

- **Main Courses**

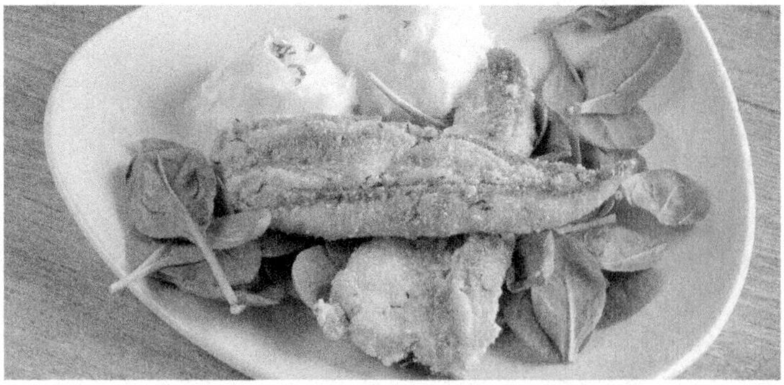

Enjoy hearty, wholesome meals with recipes like Lemon Garlic Salmon, Stuffed Bell Peppers, or Honey Mustard Chicken Thighs.

- **Sides**

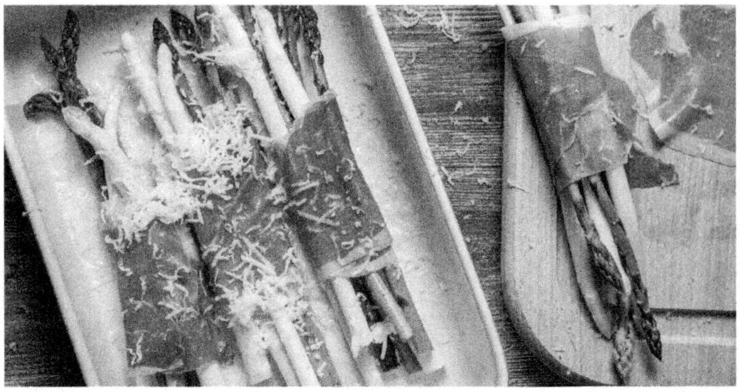

Complement your main dishes with healthy, flavorful sides like Roasted Brussels Sprouts, Garlic Parmesan Asparagus, or Curried Cauliflower.

- **Desserts**

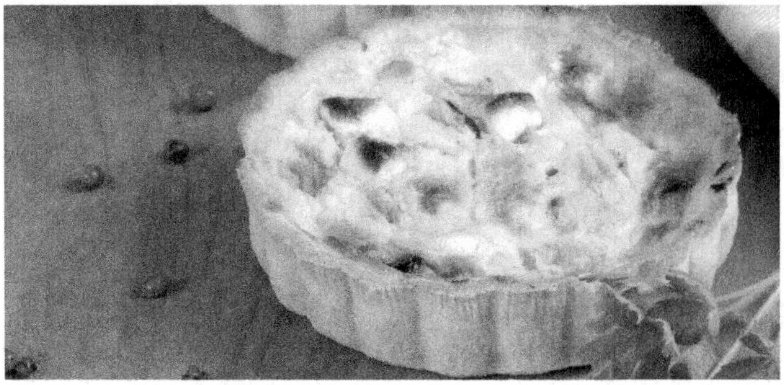

Indulge in guilt-free desserts such as Air Fried Apples, Chocolate Banana Bread, or Coconut Shrimp.

- **Vegetarian/Vegan Options**

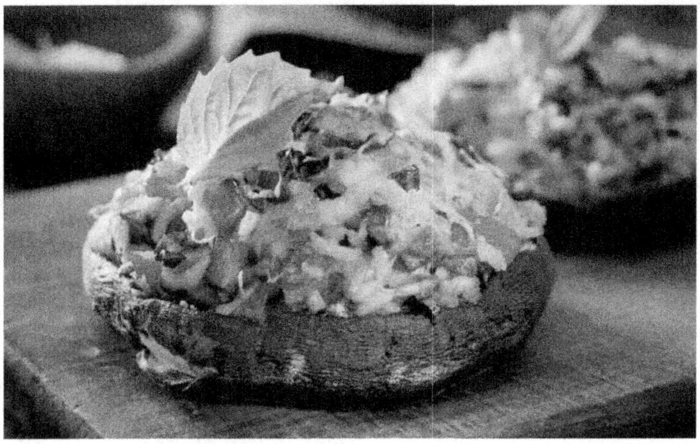

Discover a variety of plant-based dishes such as Stuffed Portobello Mushrooms, Vegan Buffalo Cauliflower Bites, and Spiced Chickpeas.

Each recipe will include easy-to-follow instructions, a clear list of ingredients, and full nutritional information to help you maintain a balanced, healthy diet. Whether you're a seasoned chef or new to the kitchen, this cookbook is designed to make healthy cooking accessible, enjoyable, and delicious.

What nutritional benefits does this cookbook provide?

The "Air Fryer Diet Cookbook" aims to support a balanced and healthy lifestyle by offering recipes that maximize the nutritional potential of ingredients and the air fryer's unique cooking capabilities.

Lower Fat Content

By utilizing the air fryer's technology, recipes in this cookbook require significantly less oil than traditional cooking methods, resulting in dishes with lower fat content.

Calorie Control

Lower fat content also means fewer calories. This cookbook can support weight management efforts and overall calorie control.

Nutrient Retention

The fast cooking times and minimal use of water in air frying help to better preserve heat-sensitive nutrients like vitamin C and certain B vitamins in your food.

Balanced Meals

The recipes are designed to offer a balance of protein, carbohydrates, and healthy fats, along with a generous serving of fruits and vegetables, to ensure you're getting a variety of nutrients necessary for overall health.

Variety

The cookbook includes a wide array of recipes, from vegetables to lean meats and legumes, ensuring you're not only enjoying a diverse diet but also consuming a wide spectrum of essential vitamins, minerals, and antioxidants.

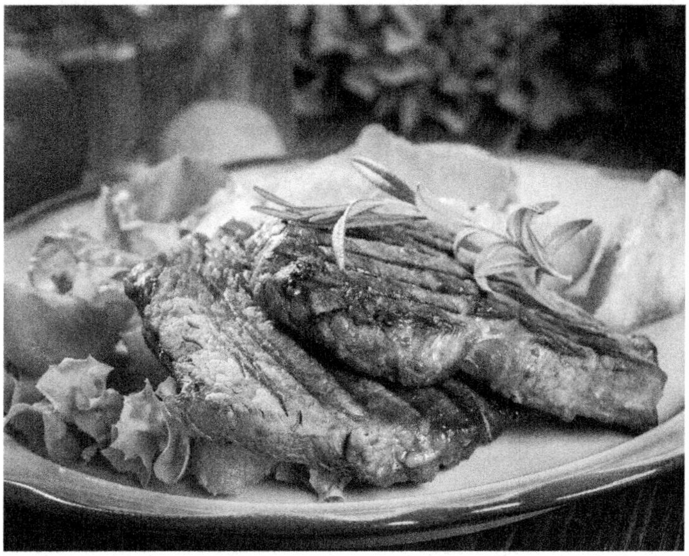

Dietary Accommodations

For those with specific dietary needs, the cookbook also includes vegetarian, vegan, and gluten-free options, among others.

Portion Control

The recipes are portioned to help prevent overeating and support healthy eating habits.

How does Air Fryer diet cookbook provide convenience for people?

- **Easy-to-Follow Recipes**

Each recipe in the cookbook is clearly written with step-by-step instructions. This makes them accessible for cooks of all skill levels, from beginners to seasoned home chefs.

- **Varied Meal Options**

The cookbook features a wide range of recipes, from breakfast, lunch, dinner, to snacks and desserts. This means you don't have to search elsewhere for air fryer recipes – it's a comprehensive, one-stop resource.

- **Efficient Cooking**

Air fryers are known for their speed and efficiency. The recipes in this cookbook are designed to make full use of this feature, helping you save time in the kitchen.

- **Nutritional Information**

Each recipe includes detailed nutritional information. This is particularly helpful for those who are tracking their caloric intake or are on specific diets.

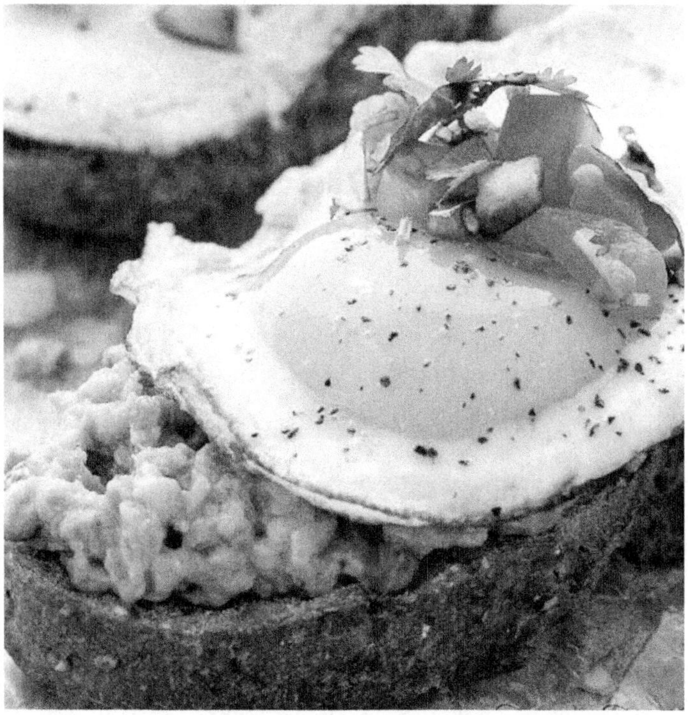

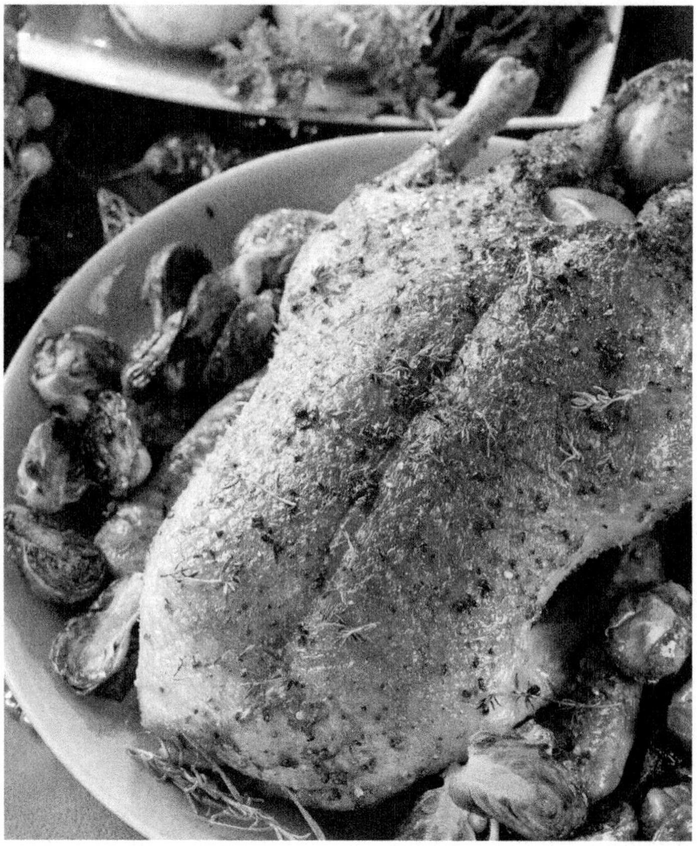

- **Shopping Lists**

The cookbook provides a list of ingredients for each recipe, making grocery shopping easier and more efficient.

- **Cooking Tips and Techniques**

In addition to the recipes, the cookbook also offers practical tips and techniques for using your air fryer, cleaning and maintaining it, and adapting recipes based on personal preferences or dietary restrictions.

- **Time-saving**

Since air fryer typically cooks faster than traditional oven or stove-top methods, using the recipes in this cookbook can significantly cut down your cooking time, giving you more freedom for other activities.

By making the cooking process simpler, more efficient, and more enjoyable, the "Air Fryer Diet Cookbook" is an excellent tool for anyone who wants to enjoy nutritious and delicious meals at home without the hassle and time commitment often associated with healthy cooking.

Measurement Conversions

BASIC KITCHEN CONVERSIONS & EQUIVALENTS

DRY MEASUREMENTS CONVERSION CHART

3 TEASPOONS = 1 TABLESPOON = 1/16 CUP

6 TEASPOONS = 2 TABLESPOONS = 1/8 CUP

12 TEASPOONS = 4 TABLESPOONS = 1/4 CUP

24 TEASPOONS = 8 TABLESPOONS = 1/2 CUP

36 TEASPOONS = 12 TABLESPOONS = 3/4 CUP

48 TEASPOONS = 16 TABLESPOONS = 1 CUP

METRIC TO US COOKING CONVERSIONS

OVEN TEMPERATURES

120 °C = 250 °F

160 °C = 320 °F

180° C = 350 °F

205 °C = 400 °F

220 °C = 425 °F

LIQUID MEASUREMENTS CONVERSION CHART

8 FLUID OUNCES = 1 CUP = 1/2 PINT = 1/4 QUART

16 FLUID OUNCES = 2 CUPS = 1 PINT = 1/2 QUART

32 FLUID OUNCES = 4 CUPS = 2 PINTS = 1 QUART

= 1/4 GALLON

128 FLUID OUNCES = 16 CUPS = 8 PINTS = 4 QUARTS = 1 GALLON

BAKING IN GRAMS

1 CUP FLOUR = 140 GRAMS

1 CUP SUGAR = 150 GRAMS

1 CUP POWDERED SUGAR = 160 GRAMS

1 CUP HEAVY CREAM = 235 GRAMS

VOLUME

1 MILLILITER = 1/5 TEASPOON

5 ML = 1 TEASPOON

15 ML = 1 TABLESPOON

240 ML = 1 CUP OR 8 FLUID OUNCES

1 LITER = 34 FL. OUNCES

WEIGHT

1 GRAM = .035 OUNCES

100 GRAMS = 3.5 OUNCES

500 GRAMS = 1.1 POUNDS

1 KILOGRAM = 35 OUNCES

US TO METRIC COOKING CONVERSIONS

1/5 TSP = 1 ML

1 TSP = 5 ML

1 TBSP = 15 ML

1 FL OUNCE = 30 ML

1 CUP = 237 ML

1 PINT (2 CUPS) = 473 ML

1 QUART (4 CUPS) = .95 LITER

1 GALLON (16 CUPS) = 3.8 LITERS

1 OZ = 28 GRAMS

1 POUND = 454 GRAMS

BUTTER

1 CUP BUTTER = 2 STICKS = 8 OUNCES = 230 GRAMS = 8 TABLESPOONS

WHAT DOES 1 CUP EQUAL

1 CUP = 8 FLUID OUNCES

1 CUP = 16 TABLESPOONS

1 CUP = 48 TEASPOONS

1 CUP = 1/2 PINT

1 CUP = 1/4 QUART

1 CUP = 1/16 GALLON

1 CUP = 240 ML

BAKING PAN CONVERSIONS

1 CUP ALL-PURPOSE FLOUR = 4.5 OZ

1 CUP ROLLED OATS = 3 OZ 1 LARGE EGG = 1.7 OZ

1 CUP BUTTER = 8 OZ 1 CUP MILK = 8 OZ

1 CUP HEAVY CREAM = 8.4 OZ

1 CUP GRANULATED SUGAR = 7.1 OZ

1 CUP PACKED BROWN SUGAR = 7.75 OZ

1 CUP VEGETABLE OIL = 7.7 OZ

1 CUP UNSIFTED POWDERED SUGAR = 4.4 OZ

BAKING PAN CONVERSIONS

9-INCH ROUND CAKE PAN = 12 CUPS

10-INCH TUBE PAN =16 CUPS

11-INCH BUNDT PAN = 12 CUPS

9-INCH SPRINGFORM PAN = 10 CUPS

9 X 5 INCH LOAF PAN = 8 CUPS

9-INCH SQUARE PAN = 8 CUPS

Breakfast & Snacks And Fries Recipes

Toad In The Hole, Breakfast Style

Servings: 4
Cooking Time:xx

Ingredients:

- 1 sheet of puff pastry (defrosted)
- 4 eggs
- 4 tbsp grated cheese (cheddar works well)
- 4 slices of cooked ham, cut into pieces
- Chopped fresh herbs of your choice

Directions:

1. Preheat your air fryer to 200°C
2. Take your pastry sheet and place it on a flat surface, cutting it into four pieces
3. Take two of the pastry sheets and place them inside your fryer, cooking for up to 8 minutes, until done
4. Remove the pastry and flatten the centre down with a spoon, to form a deep hole
5. Add a tablespoon of the cheese and a tablespoon of the ham into the hole
6. Crack one egg into the hole
7. Return the pastry to the air fryer and cook for another 6 minutes, or until the egg is done as you like it
8. Remove and allow to cool
9. Repeat the process with the rest of the pastry remaining
10. Sprinkle fresh herbs on top and serve

Easy Cheesy Scrambled Eggs

Servings: 1
Cooking Time:xx

Ingredients:

- 1 tbsp butter
- 2 eggs
- 100g grated cheese
- 2 tbsp milk
- Salt and pepper for seasoning

Directions:

1. Add the butter inside the air fryer pan and cook at 220°C until the butter has melted
2. Add the eggs and milk to a bowl and combine, seasoning to your liking
3. Pour the eggs into the butter panned cook for 3 minutes, stirring around lightly to scramble
4. Add the cheese and cook for another 2 more minutes

Blueberry & Lemon Breakfast Muffins

Servings: 12
Cooking Time:xx

Ingredients:

- 315g self raising flour
- 65g sugar
- 120ml double cream
- 2 tbsp of light cooking oil
- 2 eggs
- 125g blueberries
- The zest and juice of a lemon
- 1 tsp vanilla

Directions:

1. Take a small bowl and mix the self raising flour and sugar together
2. Take another bowl and mix together the oil, juice, eggs, cream, and vanilla
3. Add this mixture to the flour mixture and blend together
4. Add the blueberries and fold
5. You will need individual muffin holders, silicone works best. Spoon the mixture into the holders
6. Cook at 150°C for 10 minutes
7. Check at the halfway point to check they're not cooking too fast
8. Remove and allow to cool

European Pancakes

Servings: 5
Cooking Time:xx

Ingredients:

- 3 large eggs
- 130g flour
- 140ml whole milk
- 2 tbsp unsweetened apple sauce
- A pinch of salt

Directions:

1. Set your fryer to 200°C and add five ramekins inside to heat up
2. Place all your ingredients inside a blender to combine
3. Spray the ramekins with a little cooking spray
4. Pour the batter into the ramekins carefully
5. Fry for between 6-8 minutes, depending on your preference
6. Serve with your favourite toppings

Easy Air Fryer Sausage

Servings: 5
Cooking Time:xx

Ingredients:

- 5 uncooked sausages
- 1 tbsp mustard
- Salt and pepper for seasoning

Directions:

1. Line the basket of your fryer with parchment paper
2. Arrange the sausages inside the basket
3. Set to 180°C and cook for 15 minutes
4. Turn the sausages over and cook for another 5 minutes
5. Remove and cool
6. Drizzle the mustard over the top and season to your liking

Bocconcini Balls

Servings: 2
Cooking Time:xx

Ingredients:

- 70 g/½ cup plus ½ tablespoon plain/all-purpose flour (gluten-free if you wish)
- 1 egg, beaten
- 70 g/1 cup dried breadcrumbs (gluten-free if you wish; see page 9)
- 10 bocconcini

Directions:

1. Preheat the air-fryer to 200ºC/400ºF.
2. Place the flour, egg and breadcrumbs on 3 separate plates. Dip each bocconcini ball first in the flour to coat, then the egg, shaking off any excess before rolling in the breadcrumbs.
3. Add the breaded bocconcini to the preheated air-fryer and air-fry for 5 minutes (no need to turn them during cooking). Serve immediately.

Tangy Breakfast Hash

Servings: 6
Cooking Time:xx

Ingredients:

- 2 tbsp olive oil
- 2 sweet potatoes, cut into cubes
- 1 tbsp smoked paprika
- 1 tsp salt
- 1 tsp black pepper
- 2 slices of bacon, cut into small pieces

Directions:

1. Preheat your air fryer to 200ºC
2. Pour the olive oil into a large mixing bowl
3. Add the bacon, seasonings, potatoes and toss to evenly coat
4. Transfer the mixture into the air fryer and cook for 12-16 minutes
5. Stir after 10 minutes and continue to stir periodically for another 5 minutes

Morning Sausage Wraps

Servings: 8
Cooking Time:xx

Ingredients:

- 8 sausages, chopped into pieces
- 2 slices of cheddar cheese, cut into quarters
- 1 can of regular crescent roll dough
- 8 wooden skewers

Directions:

1. Take the dough and separate each one
2. Cut open the sausages evenly
3. The one of your crescent rolls and on the widest part, add a little sausage and then a little cheese
4. Roll the dough and tuck it until you form a triangle
5. Repeat this for four times and add into your air fryer
6. Cook at 190ºC for 3 minutes
7. Remove your dough and add a skewer for serving
8. Repeat with the other four pieces of dough

Swede Fries

Servings: 4
Cooking Time:xx

Ingredients:

- 1 medium swede/rutabaga
- ½ teaspoon salt
- ½ teaspoon freshly ground black pepper
- 1½ teaspoons dried thyme
- 1 tablespoon olive oil

Directions:

1. Preheat the air-fryer to 160ºC/325ºF.
2. Peel the swede/rutabaga and slice into fries about 6 x 1 cm/2½ x ½ in., then toss the fries in the salt, pepper, thyme and oil, making sure every fry is coated.
3. Tip into the preheated air-fryer in a single layer (you may need to cook them in two batches, depending on the size of your air-fryer) and air-fry for 15 minutes, shaking the drawer halfway through. Then increase the temperature to 180ºC/350ºF and cook for a further 5 minutes. Serve immediately.

Monte Cristo Breakfast Sandwich

Servings: 4
Cooking Time:xx

Ingredients:

- 1 egg
- 2 slices of sandwich bread
- 1/4 tsp vanilla extract
- 4 slices of sliced Swiss cheese
- 4 slices of sliced deli ham
- 4 slices of sliced turkey
- 1 tsp melted butter
- Powdered sugar for serving

Directions:

1. In a small bowl, mix together the egg and vanilla extract, combining well
2. Take your bread and assemble your sandwich, starting with a slice of cheese, then the ham, turkey, and then another slice of the cheese, with the other slice of bread on the top
3. Compress the sandwich a little, so it cooks better
4. Take a piece of cooking foil and brush over it with the butter
5. Take your sandwich and dip each side into the egg mixture, leaving it to one side for around half a minute
6. Place the sandwich on the foil and place it inside your fryer
7. Cook at 200ºC for around 10 minutes, before turning the sandwich over and cooking for another 8 minutes
8. Transfer your sandwich onto a plate and sprinkle with a little powdered sugar

Healthy Stuffed Peppers

Servings: 2
Cooking Time:xx
Ingredients:

- 1 large bell pepper, deseeded and cut into halves
- 1 tsp olive oil
- 4 large eggs
- Salt and pepper to taste

Directions:

1. Take your peppers and rub a little olive oil on the edges
2. Into each pepper, crack one egg and season with salt and pepper
3. You will need to insert a trivet into your air fryer to hold the peppers, and then arrange the peppers evenly
4. Set your fryer to 200°C and cook for 13 minutes
5. Once cooked, remove and serve with a little more seasoning, if required

Wholegrain Pitta Chips

Servings: 2
Cooking Time:xx
Ingredients:

- 2 round wholegrain pittas, chopped into quarters
- 1 teaspoon olive oil
- ½ teaspoon garlic salt

Directions:

1. Preheat the air-fryer to 180°C/350°F.
2. Spray or brush each pitta quarter with olive oil and sprinkle with garlic salt. Place in the preheated air-fryer and air-fry for 4 minutes, turning halfway through cooking. Serve immediately.

Blueberry Bread

Servings: 8
Cooking Time:xx
Ingredients:

- 260ml milk
- 3 eggs
- 25g protein powder
- 400g frozen blueberries
- 600g bisquick or pancake mixture

Directions:

1. Take a large mixing bowl and combine all ingredients until smooth
2. Preheat the air fryer to 250°C
3. Place the mixture into a loaf tin
4. Place the tin into the air fryer and cook for 30 minutes
5. A toothpick should come out clean if the bread is cooked

Patatas Bravas

Servings: 4
Cooking Time:xx

Ingredients:

- 300g potatoes
- 1 tsp garlic powder
- 1 tbsp avocado oil
- 1 tbsp smoked paprika
- Salt and pepper to taste

Directions:

1. Peel the potatoes and cut them into cubes
2. Bring a large saucepan of water to the boil and add the potatoes, cooking for 6 minutes
3. Strain the potatoes and place them on a piece of kitchen towel, allowing to dry
4. Take a large mixing bowl and add the garlic powder, salt, and pepper and add the avocado oil, mixing together well
5. Add the potatoes to the bowl and coat liberally
6. Place the potatoes into the basket and arrange them with space in-between
7. Set your fryer to 200°C
8. Cook the potatoes for 15 minutes, giving them a shake at the halfway point
9. Remove and serve

Healthy Breakfast Bagels

Servings: 2
Cooking Time:xx

Ingredients:

- 170g self raising flour
- 120ml plain yogurt
- 1 egg

Directions:

1. Take a large mixing bowl, combine the flour and the yogurt to create a dough
2. Cover a flat surface with a little extra flour and set the dough down
3. Create four separate and even balls
4. Roll each ball out into a rope shape and form a bagel with each
5. Take a small mixing bowl and whisk the egg
6. Brush the egg over the top of the bagel
7. Arrange the bagels inside your fryer evenly
8. Cook at 170°C for 10 minutes
9. Allow to cool before serving

Apple Crisps

Servings: 2
Cooking Time:xx
Ingredients:

- 2 apples, chopped
- 1 tsp cinnamon
- 2 tbsp brown sugar
- 1 tsp lemon juice
- 2.5 tbsp plain flour
- 3 tbsp oats
- 2 tbsp cold butter
- Pinch of salt

Directions:

1. Preheat the air fryer to 260ºC
2. Take a 5" baking dish and crease
3. Take a large bowl and combine the apples with the sugar, cinnamon and lemon juice
4. Add the mixture to the baking dish and cover with aluminium foil
5. Place in the air fryer and cook for 15 minutes
6. Open the lid and cook for another 5 minutes
7. Combine the rest of the ingredients in a food processor, until a crumble-type mixture occurs
8. Add over the top of the cooked apples
9. Cook with the lid open for another 5 minutes
10. Allow to cool a little before serving

Oozing Baked Eggs

Servings: 2
Cooking Time:xx
Ingredients:

- 4 eggs
- 140g smoked gouda cheese, cut into small pieces
- Salt and pepper to taste

Directions:

1. You will need two ramekin dishes and spray each one before using
2. Crack two eggs into each ramekin dish
3. Add half of the Gouda cheese to each dish
4. Season and place into the air fryer
5. Cook at 350ºC for 15 minutes, until the eggs are cooked as you like them

Breakfast Eggs & Spinach

Servings: 4
Cooking Time:xx
Ingredients:

- 500g wilted, fresh spinach
- 200g sliced deli ham
- 1 tbsp olive oil
- 4 eggs
- 4 tsp milk
- Salt and pepper to taste
- 1 tbsp butter for cooking

Directions:

1. Preheat your air fryer to 180ºC
2. You will need 4 small ramekin dishes, coated with a little butter
3. Arrange the wilted spinach, ham, 1 teaspoon of milk and 1 egg into each ramekin and season with a little salt and pepper
4. Place in the fryer 15 to 20 minutes, until the egg is cooked to your liking
5. Allow to cool before serving

Easy Cheese & Bacon Toasties

Servings: 2
Cooking Time:xx
Ingredients:

- 4 slices of sandwich bread
- 2 slices of cheddar cheese
- 5 slices of pre-cooked bacon
- 1 tbsp melted butter
- 2 slices of mozzarella cheese

Directions:

1. Take the bread and spread the butter onto one side of each slice
2. Place one slice of bread into the fryer basket, buttered side facing downwards
3. Place the cheddar on top, followed by the bacon, mozzarella and the other slice of bread on top, buttered side upwards
4. Set your fryer to 170ºC
5. Cook for 4 minutes and then turn over and cook for another 3 minutes
6. Serve whilst still hot

Crunchy Mexican Breakfast Wrap

Servings: 2
Cooking Time:xx
Ingredients:

- 2 large tortillas
- 2 corn tortillas
- 1 sliced jalapeño pepper
- 4 tbsp ranchero sauce
- 1 sliced avocado
- 25g cooked pinto beans

Directions:

1. Take each of your large tortillas and add the egg, jalapeño, sauce, the corn tortillas, the avocado and the pinto beans, in that order. If you want to add more sauce at this point, you can
2. Fold over your wrap to make sure that nothing escapes
3. Place each wrap into your fryer and cook at 190ºC for 6 minutes
4. Remove your wraps and place in the oven, cooking for a further 5 minutes at 180ºC, until crispy
5. Place each wrap into a frying pan and crisp a little more on a low heat, for a couple of minutes on each side

Sauces & Snack And Appetiser Recipes

Peppers With Aioli Dip

Servings: 4
Cooking Time:xx
Ingredients:

- 250g shishito peppers
- 2 tsp avocado oil
- 5 tbsp mayonnaise
- 2 tbsp lemon juice
- 1 minced clove of garlic
- 1 tbsp chopped parsley
- Salt and pepper for seasoning

Directions:

1. Take a medium bowl and combine the mayonnaise with the lemon juice, garlic, parsley and seasoning and create a smooth dip
2. Preheat the air fryer to 220ºC
3. Toss the peppers in the oil and add to the air fryer
4. Cook for 4 minutes, until the peppers are soft and blistered on the outside
5. Remove and serve with the dip

Mini Aubergine Parmesan Pizza

Servings: 8
Cooking Time:xx
Ingredients:

- 1 aubergine, cut into ½ inch slices
- Salt to taste
- 1 egg
- 1 tbsp water
- 100g bread crumbs
- 75g grated parmesan
- 6 tbsp pizza sauce
- 50g sliced olives
- 75g grated mozzarella
- Basil to garnish

Directions:

1. Preheat air fryer to 160ºC
2. Mix egg and water together and in another bowl mix the breadcrumbs and parmesan
3. Dip the aubergine in the egg then coat with the breadcrumbs
4. Place in the air fryer and cook for 10 minutes
5. Spoon pizza sauce on the aubergine, add olives and sprinkle with mozzarella
6. Cook for about 4 minutes until cheese has melted

Spring Rolls

Servings: 20
Cooking Time:xx

Ingredients:

- 160g dried rice noodles
- 1 tsp sesame oil
- 300g minced beef
- 200g frozen vegetables
- 1 onion, diced
- 3 cloves garlic, crushed
- 1 tsp soy sauce
- 1 tbsp vegetable oil
- 1 pack egg roll wrappers

Directions:

1. Soak the noodles in a bowl of water until soft
2. Add the minced beef, onion, garlic and vegetables to a pan and cook for 6 minutes
3. Remove from the heat, stir in the noodles and add the soy
4. Heat the air fryer to 175ºC
5. Add a diagonal strip of filling in each egg roll wrapper
6. Fold the top corner over the filling, fold in the two side corners
7. Brush the centre with water and roll to seal
8. Brush with vegetable oil, place in the air fryer and cook for about 8 minutes until browned

Spicy Peanuts

Servings: 8
Cooking Time:xx

Ingredients:

- 2 tbsp olive oil
- 3 tbsp seafood seasoning
- ½ tsp cayenne
- 300g raw peanuts
- Salt to taste

Directions:

1. Preheat the air fryer to 160ºC
2. Whisk together ingredients in a bowl and stir in the peanuts
3. Add to air fryer and cook for 10 minutes, shake then cook for a further 10 minutes
4. Sprinkle with salt and cook for another 5 minutes

Pepperoni Bread

Servings: 4
Cooking Time:xx
Ingredients:

- Cooking spray
- 400g pizza dough
- 200g pepperoni
- 1 tbsp dried oregano
- Ground pepper to taste
- Garlic salt to taste
- 1 tsp melted butter
- 1 tsp grated parmesan
- 50g grated mozzarella

Directions:

1. Line a baking tin with 2 inch sides with foil to fit in the air fryer
2. Spray with cooking spray
3. Preheat the air fryer to 200ºC
4. Roll the pizza dough into 1 inch balls and line the baking tin
5. Sprinkle with pepperoni, oregano, pepper and garlic salt
6. Brush with melted butter and sprinkle with parmesan
7. Place in the air fryer and cook for 15 minutes
8. Sprinkle with mozzarella and cook for another 2 minutes

Tasty Pumpkin Seeds

Servings: 2
Cooking Time:xx
Ingredients:

- 1 ¾ cups pumpkin seeds
- 2 tsp avocado oil
- 1 tsp paprika
- 1 tsp salt

Directions:

1. Preheat air fryer to 180ºC
2. Add all ingredients to a bowl and mix well
3. Place in the air fryer and cook for 35 minutes shaking frequently

Potato Patties

Servings: 12
Cooking Time:xx
Ingredients:

- 150g instant mash
- 50g peas and carrots
- 2 tbsp coriander
- 1 tbsp oil
- 100ml hot water
- ½ tsp turmeric
- ½ tsp cayenne
- ½ tsp salt
- ½ tsp cumin seeds
- ¼ tsp ground cumin

Directions:

1. Place all the ingredients in a bowl. Mix well cover and stand for 10 minutes
2. Preheat the air fryer to 200ºC
3. Spray the air fryer with cooking spray
4. Make 12 patties, place in the air fryer and cook for 10 minutes

Popcorn Tofu

Servings: 4
Cooking Time:xx
Ingredients:

- 400g firm tofu
- 100g chickpea flour
- 100g oatmeal
- 2 tbsp yeast
- 150ml milk
- 400g breadcrumbs
- 1 tsp garlic powder
- 1 tsp onion powder
- 1 tbsp dijon mustard
- ½ tsp salt
- ½ tsp pepper
- 2 tbsp vegetable bouillon

Directions:

1. Rip the tofu into pieces. Place the breadcrumbs into a bowl, in another bowl mix the remaining ingredients
2. Dip the tofu into the batter mix and then dip into the breadcrumbs
3. Heat the air fryer to 175°C
4. Place the tofu in the air fryer and cook for 12 minutes shaking halfway through

Roasted Almonds

Servings: 2
Cooking Time:xx
Ingredients:

- 1 tbsp soy sauce
- 1 tbsp garlic powder
- 1 tsp paprika
- ¼ tsp pepper
- 400g raw almonds

Directions:

1. Place all of the ingredients apart from the almonds in a bowl and mix
2. Add the almonds and coat well
3. Place the almonds in the air fryer and cook at 160°C for 6 minutes shaking every 2 minutes

Salt And Vinegar Chips

Servings: 4
Cooking Time:xx
Ingredients:

- 6-10 Jerusalem artichokes, thinly sliced
- 150ml apple cider vinegar
- 2 tbsp olive oil
- Sea salt

Directions:

1. Soak the artichoke in apple cider vinegar for 20-30 minutes
2. Preheat the air fryer to 200°C
3. Coat the artichoke in olive oil
4. Place in the air fryer and cook for 15 Minutes
5. Sprinkle with salt

Sweet Potato Crisps

Servings: 4
Cooking Time:xx

Ingredients:

- 1 sweet potato, peeled and thinly sliced
- 2 tbsp oil
- ¼ tsp salt
- ¼ tsp pepper
- 1 tsp chopped rosemary
- Cooking spray

Directions:

1. Place all ingredients in a bowl and mix well
2. Place in the air fryer and cook at 175ºC for about 15 minutes until crispy

Lumpia

Servings: 16
Cooking Time:xx

Ingredients:

- 400g Italian sausage
- 1 sliced onion
- 1 chopped carrot
- 50g chopped water chestnuts
- Cooking spray
- 2 cloves minced, garlic
- 2 tbsp soy sauce
- ½ tsp salt
- ¼ tsp ground ginger
- 16 spring roll wrappers

Directions:

1. Cook sausage in a pan for about 5 minutes. Add green onions, onions, water chestnuts and carrot cook for 7 minutes
2. Add garlic and cook for a further 2 minutes
3. Add the soy sauce, salt and ginger, stir to mix well
4. Add filling to each spring roll wrapper.
5. Roll over the bottom and tuck in the sides, continue to roll up the spring roll
6. Spray with cooking spray and place in the air fryer
7. Cook at 200ºC for 4 minutes turn and cook for a further 4 minutes

Pork Jerky

Servings: 35
Cooking Time:xx

Ingredients:

- 300g mince pork
- 1 tbsp oil
- 1 tbsp sriracha
- 1 tbsp soy
- ½ tsp pink curing salt
- 1 tbsp rice vinegar
- ½ tsp salt
- ½ tsp pepper
- ½ tsp onion powder

Directions:

1. Mix all ingredients in a bowl until combined
2. Refrigerate for about 8 hours
3. Shape into sticks and place in the air fryer
4. Heat the air fryer to 160ºC
5. Cook for 1 hour turn then cook for another hour
6. Turn again and cook for another hour
7. Cover with paper and sit for 8 hours

Cheese Wontons

Servings: 8
Cooking Time:xx

Ingredients:

- 8 wonton wrappers
- 1 carton pimento cheese
- Small dish of water
- Cooking spray

Directions:

1. Place one tsp of cheese in the middle of each wonton wrapper
2. Brush the edges of each wonton wrapper with water
3. Fold over to create a triangle and seal
4. Heat the air fryer to 190ºC
5. Spray the wontons with cooking spray
6. Place in the air fryer and cook for 3 minutes
7. Turnover and cook for a further 3 minutes

Corn Nuts

Servings: 8
Cooking Time:xx

Ingredients:

- 1 giant white corn
- 3 tbsp vegetable oil
- 2 tsp salt

Directions:

1. Place the corn in a large bowl, cover with water and sit for 8 hours
2. Drain, pat dry and air dry for 20 minutes
3. Preheat the air fryer to 200ºC
4. Place in a bowl and coat with oil and salt
5. Cook in the air fryer for 10 minutes shake then cook for a further 10 minutes

Salt And Vinegar Chickpeas

Servings: 5
Cooking Time:xx

Ingredients:

- 1 can chickpeas
- 100ml white vinegar
- 1 tbsp olive oil
- Salt to taste

Directions:

1. Combine chickpeas and vinegar in a pan, simmer remove from heat and stand for 30 minutes
2. Preheat the air fryer to 190ºC
3. Drain chickpeas
4. Place chickpeas in the air fryer and cook for about 4 minutes
5. Pour chickpeas into an ovenproof bowl drizzle with oil, sprinkle with salt
6. Place bowl in the air fryer and cook for another 4 minutes

Garlic Cheese Bread

Servings: 2
Cooking Time:xx

Ingredients:

- 250g grated mozzarella
- 50g grated parmesan
- 1 egg
- ½ tsp garlic powder

Directions:

1. Line air fryer with parchment paper
2. Mix ingredients in a bowl
3. Press into a circle onto the parchment paper in the air fryer
4. Heat the air fryer to 175ºC
5. Cook for 10 minutes

Snack Style Falafel

Servings: 15
Cooking Time:xx

Ingredients:

- 150g dry garbanzo beans
- 300g coriander
- 75g flat leaf parsley
- 1 red onion, quartered
- 1 clove garlic
- 2 tbsp chickpea flour
- Cooking spray
- 1 tbsp cumin
- 1 tbsp coriander
- 1 tbsp sriracha
- ½ tsp baking powder
- Salt and pepper to taste
- ¼ tsp baking soda

Directions:

1. Add all ingredients apart from the baking soda and baking powder to a food processor and blend well
2. Cover and rest for 1 hour
3. Heat air fryer to 190ºC
4. Add baking powder and baking soda to mix and combine
5. Form mix into 15 equal balls
6. Spray air fryer with cooking spray
7. Add to air fryer and cook for 8-10 minutes

Tostones

Servings: 4
Cooking Time:xx

Ingredients:

- 2 unripe plantains
- Olive oil cooking spray
- 300ml of water
- Salt to taste

Directions:

1. Preheat the air fryer to 200°C
2. Slice the tips off the plantain
3. Cut the plantain into 1 inch chunks
4. Place in the air fryer spray with oil and cook for 5 minutes
5. Remove the plantain from the air fryer and smash to ½ inch pieces
6. Soak in a bowl of salted water
7. Remove from the water and return to the air fryer season with salt cook for 5 minutes
8. Turn and cook for another 5 minutes

Garlic Pizza Toast

Servings: 8
Cooking Time:xx

Ingredients:

- 1 pack garlic Texas toast, or 8 slices of bread topped with garlic butter
- 100g pizza sauce
- 50g pepperoni
- 100g grated cheese

Directions:

1. Top each piece of toast with pizza sauce
2. Add cheese and pepperoni
3. Heat air fryer to 190°C
4. Place in the air fryer and cook for 5 minutes

Poultry Recipes

Honey Cajun Chicken Thighs

Servings: 6
Cooking Time:xx
Ingredients:

- 100ml buttermilk
- 1 tsp hot sauce
- 400g skinless, boneless chicken thighs
- 150g all purpose flour
- 60g tapioca flour
- 2.5 tsp cajun seasoning
- ½ tsp garlic salt
- ½ tsp honey powder
- ¼ tsp ground paprika
- ⅛ tsp cayenne pepper
- 4 tsp honey

Directions:

1. Take a large bowl and combine the buttermilk and hot sauce
2. Transfer to a plastic bag and add the chicken thighs
3. Allow to marinate for 30 minutes
4. Take another bowl and add the flour, tapioca flour, cajun seasoning, garlic, salt, honey powder, paprika, and cayenne pepper, combining well
5. Dredge the chicken through the mixture
6. Preheat the air fryer to 175C
7. Cook for 15 minutes before flipping the thighs over and cooking for another 10 minutes
8. Drizzle 1 tsp of honey over each thigh

Air Fryer Bbq Chicken

Servings: 4
Cooking Time:xx
Ingredients:

- 1 whole chicken
- 2 tbsp avocado oil
- 1 tbsp kosher salt
- 1 tsp ground pepper
- 1 tsp garlic powder
- 1 tsp paprika
- ½ tsp dried basil
- ½ tsp dried oregano
- ½ tsp dried thyme

Directions:

1. Mix the seasonings together and spread over chicken
2. Place the chicken in the air fryer breast side down
3. Cook at 182C for 50 minutes and then breast side up for 10 minutes
4. Carve and serve

Buffalo Chicken Wontons

Servings: 6
Cooking Time:xx
Ingredients:

- 200g shredded chicken
- 1 tbsp buffalo sauce
- 4 tbsp softened cream cheese
- 1 sliced spring onion
- 2 tbsp blue cheese crumbles
- 12 wonton wrappers

Directions:

1. Preheat the air fryer to 200°C
2. Take a bowl and combine the chicken and buffalo sauce
3. In another bowl mix the cream cheese until a smooth consistency has formed and then combine the scallion blue cheese and seasoned chicken
4. Take the wonton wrappers and run wet fingers along each edge
5. Place 1 tbsp of the filling into the centre of the wonton and fold the corners together
6. Cook at 200°C for 3 to 5 minutes, until golden brown

Keto Tandoori Chicken

Servings: 2
Cooking Time:xx
Ingredients:

- 500g chicken tenders, halved
- 1 tbsp minced ginger
- 1 tbsp minced garlic
- 1 tsp cayenne pepper
- 1 tsp turmeric
- 1 tsp garam masala
- 60ml yogurt
- 25g coriander leaves
- Salt and pepper to taste

Directions:

1. Take a large mixing bowl and combine all the ingredients, except the chicken
2. Once combined, add the chicken to the bowl and make sure it is fully coated
3. Preheat the air fryer to 160°C
4. Place the chicken in the air fryer and baste with oil
5. Cook for 10 minutes, turning over and then cooking for another 5 minutes
6. Serve whilst still warm

Hawaiian Chicken

Servings: 2
Cooking Time:xx

Ingredients:

- 2 chicken breasts
- 1 tbsp butter
- A pinch of salt and pepper
- 160ml pineapple juice
- 25g brown sugar
- 3 tbsp soy sauce
- 2 tsp water
- 1 clove of garlic, minced
- 1 tsp grated ginger
- 2 tsp cornstarch

Directions:

1. Preheat the air fryer to 260°C
2. Take a bowl and combine the butter and salt and pepper
3. Cover the chicken with the butter and cook in the fryer for 15 minutes, turning halfway
4. Remove and allow to rest for 5 minutes
5. Take another bowl and mix together the pineapple juice, soy sauce, garlic, ginger, and brown sugar
6. Transfer to a saucepan and simmer for 5 minutes
7. Combine the water and cornstarch and add to the sauce, stirring continually for another minute
8. Slice the chicken into strips and pour the sauce over the top

Buffalo Wings

Servings: 4
Cooking Time:xx

Ingredients:

- 500g chicken wings
- 1 tbsp olive oil
- 5 tbsp cayenne pepper sauce
- 75g butter
- 2 tbsp vinegar
- 1 tsp garlic powder
- ¼ tsp cayenne pepper

Directions:

1. Preheat the air fryer to 182C
2. Take a large mixing bowl and add the chicken wings
3. Drizzle oil over the wings, coating evenly
4. Cook for 25 minutes and then flip the wings and cook for 5 more minutes
5. In a saucepan over a medium heat, mix the hot pepper sauce, butter, vinegar, garlic powder and cayenne pepper, combining well
6. Pour the sauce over the wings and flip to coat, before serving

Grain-free Chicken Katsu

Servings: 4
Cooking Time:xx

Ingredients:

- 125 g/1¼ cups ground almonds
- ½ teaspoon salt
- ½ teaspoon garlic powder
- ½ teaspoon dried parsley
- ½ teaspoon freshly ground black pepper
- ¼ teaspoon onion powder
- ¼ teaspoon dried oregano
- 450 g/1 lb. mini chicken fillets
- 1 egg, beaten
- oil, for spraying/drizzling
- coriander/cilantro leaves, to serve
- KATSU SAUCE
- 1 teaspoon olive oil or avocado oil
- 1 courgette/zucchini (approx. 150 g/5 oz.), finely chopped
- 1 carrot (approx. 100 g/3½ oz.), finely chopped
- 1 onion (approx. 120 g/4½ oz.), finely chopped
- 1 eating apple (approx. 150 g/5 oz.), cored and finely chopped
- 1 teaspoon ground ginger
- 1 teaspoon ground turmeric
- 2 teaspoons ground cumin
- 2 teaspoons ground coriander
- 1½ teaspoons mild chilli/chili powder
- 1 teaspoon garlic powder
- 1½ tablespoons runny honey
- 1 tablespoon soy sauce (gluten-free if you wish)
- 700 ml/3 cups vegetable stock (700 ml/3 cups water with 1½ stock cubes)

Directions:

1. First make the sauce. The easiest way to ensure all the vegetables and apple are finely chopped is to combine them in a food processor. Heat the oil in a large saucepan and sauté the finely chopped vegetables and apple for 5 minutes. Add all the seasonings, honey, soy sauce and stock and stir well, then bring to a simmer and simmer for 30 minutes.
2. Meanwhile, mix together the ground almonds, seasonings and spices. Dip each chicken fillet into the beaten egg, then into the almond-spice mix, making sure each fillet is fully coated. Spray the coated chicken fillets with olive oil (or simply drizzle over).
3. Preheat the air-fryer to 180ºC/350ºF.
4. Place the chicken fillets in the preheated air-fryer and air-fry for 10 minutes, turning halfway through cooking. Check the internal temperature of the chicken has reached at least 74ºC/165ºF using a meat thermometer – if not, cook for another few minutes.
5. Blend the cooked sauce in a food processor until smooth. Serve the chicken with the Katsu Sauce drizzled over (if necessary, reheat the sauce gently before serving) and scattered with coriander leaves. Any unused sauce can be frozen.

Chicken Fried Rice

Servings: 4
Cooking Time:xx

Ingredients:

- 400g cooked white rice
- 400g cooked chicken, diced
- 200g frozen peas and carrots
- 6 tbsp soy sauce
- 1 tbsp vegetable oil
- 1 diced onion

Directions:

1. Take a large bowl and add the rice, vegetable oil and soy sauce and combine well
2. Add the frozen peas, carrots, diced onion and the chicken and mix together well
3. Pour the mixture into a nonstick pan
4. Place the pan into the air fryer
5. Cook at 182C for 20 minutes

Smoky Chicken Breast

Servings: 2
Cooking Time:xx

Ingredients:

- 2 halved chicken breasts
- 2 tsp olive oil
- 1 tsp ground thyme
- 2 tsp paprika
- 1tsp cumin
- 0.5 tsp cayenne pepper
- 0.5 tsp onion powder
- Salt and pepper to taste

Directions:

1. In a medium bowl, combine the spices together
2. Pour the spice mixture onto a plate
3. Take each chicken breast and coat in the spices, pressing down to ensure an even distribution
4. Place the chicken to one side for 5 minutes
5. Preheat your air fryer to 180ºC
6. Arrange the chicken inside the fryer and cook for 10 minutes
7. Turn the chicken over and cook for another 10 minutes
8. Remove from the fryer and allow to sit for 5 minutes before serving

Chicken And Wheat Stir Fry

Servings: 4
Cooking Time:xx

Ingredients:

- 1 onion
- 1 clove of garlic
- 200g skinless boneless chicken breast halves
- 3 whole tomatoes
- 400ml water
- 1 chicken stock cube
- 1 tbsp curry powder
- 130g wheat berries
- 1 tbsp vegetable oil

Directions:

1. Thinly slice the onion and garlic
2. Chop the chicken and tomatoes into cubes
3. Take a large saucepan and add the water, chicken stock, curry powder and wheat berries, combining well
4. Pour the oil into the air fryer bowl and heat for 5 minutes at 200ºC
5. Add the remaining ingredients and pour the contents into the air fryer
6. Cook for 15 minutes

Orange Chicken

Servings: 2
Cooking Time:xx

Ingredients:

- 600g chicken thighs, boneless and skinless
- 2 tbsp cornstarch
- 60ml orange juice
- 1 tbsp soy sauce
- 2 tbsp brown sugar
- 1 tbsp rice wine vinegar
- 1/4 teaspoon ground ginger
- Pinch of red pepper flakes
- Zest of one orange
- 2 tsp water and 2 tsp cornstarch mixed together

Directions:

1. Preheat your air fryer to 250°C
2. Take a bowl and combine the chicken with the cornstarch
3. Place in the air fryer and cook for 9 minutes
4. Take a bowl and combine the rest of the ingredients, except for the water and cornstarch mixture
5. Place in a saucepan and bring to the boil and then turn down to a simmer for 5 minutes
6. Add the water and cornstarch mixture to the pan and combine well
7. Remove the chicken from the fryer and pour the sauce over the top

Chicken Balls, Greek-style

Servings: 4
Cooking Time:xx

Ingredients:

- 500g ground chicken
- 1 egg
- 1 tbsp dried oregano
- 1.5 tbsp garlic paste
- 1 tsp lemon zest
- 1 tsp dried onion powder
- Salt and pepper to taste

Directions:

1. Take a bowl and combine all ingredients well
2. Use your hands to create meatballs - you should be able to make 12 balls
3. Preheat your air fryer to 260°C
4. Add the meatballs to the fryer and cook for 9 minutes

Charred Chicken Breasts

Servings: 2
Cooking Time:xx

Ingredients:

- 2 tsp paprika
- 1 tsp ground thyme
- 1 tsp cumin
- ½ tsp cayenne pepper
- ½ tsp onion powder
- ½ tsp black pepper
- ¼ tsp salt
- 2 tsp vegetable oil
- 2 skinless boneless chicken breasts, cut into halves

Directions:

1. Take a bowl and add the paprika, thyme, cumin, cayenne pepper, onion powder, black pepper and salt
2. Coat each chicken breast with oil and dredge chicken in the spice mixture
3. Preheat air fryer to 175C
4. Cook for 10 minutes and flip
5. Cook for 10 more minutes

Chicken Parmesan With Marinara Sauce

Servings: 4
Cooking Time:xx

Ingredients:

- 400g chicken breasts, sliced in half
- 250g panko breadcrumbs
- 140g grated parmesan cheese
- 140g grated mozzarella cheese
- 3 egg whites
- 200g marinara sauce
- 2 tsp Italian seasoning
- Salt and pepper to taste
- Cooking spray

Directions:

1. Preheat the air fryer to 200ºC
2. Lay the chicken slices on the work surface and pound with a mallet or a rolling pin to flatten
3. Take a mixing bowl and add the panko breadcrumbs, cheese and the seasoning, combining well
4. Add the egg whites into a separate bowl
5. Dip the chicken into the egg whites and then the breadcrumbs
6. Cook for 7 minutes in the air fryer

Healthy Bang Bang Chicken

Servings: 4
Cooking Time:xx
Ingredients:

- 500g chicken breasts, cut into pieces of around 1" in size
- 1 beaten egg
- 50ml milk
- 1 tbsp hot pepper sauce
- 80g flour
- 70g tapioca starch
- 1 ½ tsp seasoned starch
- 1 tsp garlic granules
- ½ tsp cumin
- 6 tbsp plain Greek yogurt
- 3 tbsp sweet chilli sauce
- 1 tsp hot sauce

Directions:

1. Preheat the air fryer to 190°C
2. Take a mixing bowl and combine the egg, milk and hot sauce
3. Take another bowl and combine the flour, tapioca starch, salt, garlic and cumin
4. Dip the chicken pieces into the sauce bowl and then into the flour bowl
5. Place the chicken into the air fryer
6. Whilst cooking, mix together the Greek yogurt, sweet chilli sauce and hot sauce and serve with the chicken

Bacon Wrapped Chicken Thighs

Servings: 4
Cooking Time:xx
Ingredients:

- 75g softened butter
- ½ clove minced garlic
- ¼ tsp dried thyme
- ¼ tsp dried basil
- ⅛ tsp coarse salt
- 100g thick cut bacon
- 350g chicken thighs, boneless and skinless
- 2 tsp minced garlic
- Salt and pepper to taste

Directions:

1. Take a mixing bowl and add the softened butter, garlic, thyme, basil, salt and pepper, combining well
2. Place the butter onto a sheet of plastic wrap and roll up to make a butter log
3. Refrigerate for about 2 hours
4. Remove the plastic wrap
5. Place one bacon strip onto the butter and then place the chicken thighs on top of the bacon. Sprinkle with garlic
6. Place the cold butter into the middle of the chicken thigh and tuck one end of bacon into the chicken
7. Next, fold over the chicken thigh whilst rolling the bacon around
8. Repeat with the rest
9. Preheat the air fryer to 188C
10. Cook the chicken until white in the centre and the juices run clear

Olive Stained Turkey Breast

Servings: 14
Cooking Time:xx

Ingredients:

- The brine from a can of olives
- 150ml buttermilk
- 300g boneless and skinless turkey breasts
- 1 sprig fresh rosemary
- 2 sprigs fresh thyme

Directions:

1. Take a mixing bowl and combine the olive brine and buttermilk
2. Pour the mixture over the turkey breast
3. Add the rosemary and thyme sprigs
4. Place into the refrigerator for 8 hours
5. Remove from the fridge and let the turkey reach room temperature
6. Preheat the air fryer to 175C
7. Cook for 15 minutes, ensuring the turkey is cooked through before serving

Pepper & Lemon Chicken Wings

Servings: 2
Cooking Time:xx

Ingredients:

- 1kg chicken wings
- 1/4 tsp cayenne pepper
- 2 tsp lemon pepper seasoning
- 3 tbsp butter
- 1 tsp honey
- An extra 1 tsp lemon pepper seasoning for the sauce

Directions:

1. Preheat the air fryer to 260ºC
2. Place the lemon pepper seasoning and cayenne in a bowl and combine
3. Coat the chicken in the seasoning
4. Place the chicken in the air fryer and cook for 20 minutes, turning over halfway
5. Turn the temperature up to 300ºC and cook for another 6 minutes
6. Meanwhile, melt the butter and combine with the honey and the rest of the seasoning
7. Remove the wings from the air fryer and pour the sauce over the top

Quick Chicken Nuggets

Servings: 4
Cooking Time:xx

Ingredients:

- 500g chicken tenders
- 25g ranch salad dressing mixture
- 2 tbsp plain flour
- 100g breadcrumbs
- 1 egg, beaten
- Olive oil spray

Directions:

1. Take a large mixing bowl and arrange the chicken inside
2. Sprinkle the seasoning over the top and ensure the chicken is evenly coated
3. Place the chicken to one side for around 10 minutes
4. Add the flour into a resealable bag
5. Crack the egg into a small mixing bowl and whisk
6. Pour the breadcrumbs onto a medium sized plate
7. Transfer the chicken into the resealable bag and coat with the flour, giving it a good shake
8. Remove the chicken and dip into the egg, and then rolling it into the breadcrumbs, coating evenly
9. Repeat with all pieces of the chicken
10. Heat your air fryer to 200ºC
11. Arrange the chicken inside the fryer and add a little olive oil spray to avoid sticking
12. Cook for 4 minutes, before turning over and cooking for another 4 minutes
13. Remove and serve whilst hot

Turkey And Mushroom Burgers

Servings: 2
Cooking Time:xx

Ingredients:

- 180g mushrooms
- 500g minced turkey
- 1 tbsp of your favourite chicken seasoning, e.g. Maggi
- 1 tsp onion powder
- 1 tsp garlic powder
- Salt and pepper to taste

Directions:

1. Place the mushrooms in a food processor and puree
2. Add all the seasonings and mix well
3. Remove from the food processor and transfer to a mixing bowl
4. Add the minced turkey and combine again
5. Shape the mix into 5 burger patties
6. Spray with cooking spray and place in the air fryer
7. Cook at 160ºC for 10 minutes, until cooked.

Beef & Lamb And Pork Recipes

Mongolian Beef

Servings: 4
Cooking Time:xx

Ingredients:

- 500g steak
- 25g cornstarch
- 2 tsp vegetable oil
- ½ tsp ginger
- 1 tbsp garlic minced
- 75g soy sauce
- 75g water
- 100g brown sugar

Directions:

1. Slice the steak and coat in corn starch
2. Place in the air fryer and cook at 200°C for 10 minutes turning halfway
3. Place remaining ingredients in a sauce pan and gently warm
4. When cooked place the steak in a bowl and pour the sauce over

Sticky Asian Beef

Servings: 2
Cooking Time:xx

Ingredients:

- 1 tbsp coconut oil
- 2 sliced peppers
- 25g liquid aminos
- 25g cup water
- 100g brown sugar
- ¼ tsp pepper
- ½ tsp ground ginger
- ½ tbsp minced garlic
- 1 tsp red pepper flakes
- 600g steak thinly sliced
- ¼ tsp salt

Directions:

1. Melt the coconut oil in a pan, add the peppers and cook until softened
2. In another pan add the aminos, brown sugar, ginger, garlic and pepper flakes. Mix and bring to the boil, simmer for 10 mins
3. Season the steak with salt and pepper
4. Put the steak in the air fryer and cook at 200°C for 10 minutes. Turn the steak and cook for a further 5 minutes until crispy
5. Add the steak to the peppers then mix with the sauce
6. Serve with rice

Salt And Pepper Belly Pork

Servings: 4
Cooking Time:xx

Ingredients:

- 500g belly pork
- 1 tsp pepper
- ½ tsp salt

Directions:

1. Cut the pork into bite size pieces and season with salt and pepper
2. Heat the air fryer to 200°C
3. Place in the air fryer and cook for 15 minutes until crisp

Breaded Bone-in Pork Chops

Servings: 2
Cooking Time:xx

Ingredients:

- 2 pork chops with the bone in
- 250g Italian breadcrumbs
- 2 tbsp mayonnaise
- 1/2 tsp garlic powder
- 1/2 tsp onion powder
- 1/2 tsp thyme
- 1/2 tsp paprika
- Salt and pepper to taste

Directions:

1. Preheat the air fryer to 260°C
2. Take a large bowl and add the breadcrumbs, garlic powder, paprika, salt and pepper, and thyme, and onion powder, combining well
3. Cover the pork chops with the mayonnaise making sure to cover both sides
4. Coat the meat with the seasoning mixture, making sure it is fully covered
5. Cook the pork chops in the fryer for 10 minutes, turning over halfway

Meatballs In Tomato Sauce

Servings: 4
Cooking Time:xx

Ingredients:

- 1 small onion
- 300g minced pork
- 1 tbsp chopped parsley
- 1 tbsp thyme
- 1 egg
- 3 tbsp bread crumbs
- Salt and pepper to taste

Directions:

1. Place all ingredients into a bowl and mix well
2. Shape mixture into 12 meatballs
3. Heat the air fryer to 200°C
4. Place the meatballs into the air fryer and cook for about 7 minutes
5. Tip the meatballs into an oven dish add the tomato sauce and cook for about 5 minutes in the air fryer until warmed through

Pork Taquitos

Servings: 5
Cooking Time:xx
Ingredients:

- 400g shredded pork
- 500g grated mozzarella
- 10 flour tortillas
- The juice of 1 lime
- Cooking spray

Directions:

1. Preheat air fryer to 190°C
2. Sprinkle lime juice on the pork and mix
3. Microwave tortilla for about 10 seconds to soften
4. Add a little pork and cheese to a tortilla
5. Roll then tortilla up, and place in the air fryer
6. Cook for about 7 minutes until golden, turn halfway through cooking

Beef Nacho Pinwheels

Servings: 6
Cooking Time:xx
Ingredients:

- 500g minced beef
- 1 packet of taco seasoning
- 300ml water
- 300ml sour cream
- 6 tostadas
- 6 flour tortillas
- 3 tomatoes
- 250g nacho cheese
- 250g shredded lettuce
- 250g Mexican cheese

Directions:

1. Preheat air fryer to 200°C
2. Brown the mince in a pan and add the taco seasoning
3. Share the remaining ingredients between the tortillas
4. Fold the edges of the tortillas up towards the centre, should look like a pinwheel
5. Lay seam down in the air fryer and cook for 2 minutes
6. Turnover and cook for a further 2 minutes

Sweet And Sticky Ribs

Servings:2
Cooking Time:1 Hour 15 Minutes
Ingredients:

- 500 g / 17.6 oz pork ribs
- 2 cloves garlic, minced
- 2 tbsp soy sauce
- 2 tsp honey
- 1 tbsp cayenne pepper
- 1 tsp olive oil
- 2 tbsp BBQ sauce
- 1 tsp salt
- 1 tsp black pepper

Directions:

1. Place the pork ribs on a clean surface and cut them into smaller chunks if necessary.
2. In a small mixing bowl, combine the minced garlic, soy sauce, 1 tsp honey, cayenne pepper, olive oil, BBQ sauce, salt, and pepper. Rub the pork ribs into the sauce and spice the mixture until fully coated.
3. Place the coated ribs in the fridge for 1 hour. Meanwhile, preheat the air fryer to 180 °C / 350 °F and line the bottom of the basket with parchment paper.
4. After one hour, transfer the pork ribs into the prepared air fryer basket. Close the lid and cook for 15 minutes, using tongs to turn them halfway through.
5. Once cooked, remove the ribs from the air fryer and use a brush to top each rib with the remaining 1 tsp honey.
6. Return the ribs to the air fryer for a further 2-3 minutes to heat the honey glaze before serving.

Bbq Ribs

Servings: 2
Cooking Time:xx
Ingredients:

- 500g ribs
- 3 chopped garlic cloves
- 4 tbsp bbq sauce
- 1 tbsp honey
- ½ tsp five spice
- 1 tsp sesame oil
- 1 tsp salt
- 1 tsp black pepper
- 1 tsp soy sauce

Directions:

1. Chop the ribs into small pieces and place them in a bowl
2. Add all the ingredients into the bowl and mix well
3. Marinate for 4 hours
4. Preheat the air fryer to 180ºC
5. Place the ribs into the air fryer and cook for 15 minutes
6. Coat the ribs in honey and cook for a further 15 minutes

Fillet Mignon Wrapped In Bacon

Servings: 2
Cooking Time:xx

Ingredients:

- 1 kg filet mignon
- 500g bacon slices
- Olive oil

Directions:

1. Wrap the fillets in bacon
2. Season with salt and pepper and brush with olive oil
3. Place in the air fryer cook at 200°C for 9 minutes turning halfway through

Pork Chops With Raspberry And Balsamic

Servings: 4
Cooking Time:xx

Ingredients:

- 2 large eggs
- 30ml milk
- 250g panko bread crumbs
- 250g finely chopped pecans
- 1 tbsp orange juice
- 4 pork chops
- 30ml balsamic vinegar
- 2 tbsp brown sugar
- 2 tbsp raspberry jam

Directions:

1. Preheat air fryer to 200°C
2. Mix the eggs and milk together in a bowl
3. In another bowl mix the breadcrumbs and pecans
4. Coat the pork chops in flour, egg and then coat in the breadcrumbs
5. Place in the air fryer and cook for 12 minutes until golden turning halfway
6. Put the remaining ingredients in a pan simmer for about 6 minutes, serve with the pork chops

Honey & Mustard Meatballs

Servings: 4
Cooking Time:xx

Ingredients:

- 500g minced pork
- 1 red onion
- 1 tsp mustard
- 2 tsp honey
- 1 tsp garlic puree
- 1 tsp pork seasoning
- Salt and pepper

Directions:

1. Thinly slice the onion
2. Place all the ingredients in a bowl and mix until well combined
3. Form into meatballs, place in the air fryer and cook at 180°C for 10 minutes

Japanese Pork Chops

Servings: 4
Cooking Time:xx

Ingredients:

- 6 boneless pork chops
- 30g flour
- 2 beaten eggs
- 2 tbsp sweet chilli sauce
- 500g cup seasoned breadcrumbs
- ⅛ tsp salt
- ⅛ tsp pepper
- Tonkatsu sauce to taste

Directions:

1. Place the flour, breadcrumbs and eggs in 3 separate bowls
2. Sprinkle both sides of the pork with salt and pepper
3. Coat the pork in flour, egg and then breadcrumbs
4. Place in the air fryer and cook at 180°C for 8 minutes, turn then cook for a further 5 minutes
5. Serve with sauces on the side

Cheesy Meatball Sub

Servings: 2
Cooking Time:xx

Ingredients:

- 8 frozen pork meatballs
- 5 tbsp marinara sauce
- 160g grated parmesan cheese
- 2 sub rolls or hotdog rolls
- 1/4 tsp dried oregano

Directions:

1. Preheat the air fryer to 220°C
2. Place the meatball in the air fryer and cook for around 10 minutes, turning halfway through
3. Place the marinara sauce in a bowl
4. Add the meatballs to the sauce and coat completely
5. Add the oregano on top and coat once more
6. Take the bread roll and add the mixture inside
7. Top with the cheese
8. Place the meatball sub back in the air fryer and cook for 2 minutes until the bad is toasted and the cheese has melted

Meatloaf

Servings: 2
Cooking Time:xx

Ingredients:

- 500g minced pork
- 1 egg
- 3 tbsp breadcrumbs
- 2 mushrooms thickly sliced
- 1 tbsp olive oil
- 1 chopped onion
- 1 tbsp chopped thyme
- 1 tsp salt
- Ground black pepper

Directions:

1. Preheat air fryer to 200°C
2. Combine all the ingredients in a bowl
3. Put the mix into a pan and press down firmly, coat with olive oil
4. Place pan in the air fryer and cook for 25 minutes

Beef Bulgogi Burgers

Servings: 4
Cooking Time:xx
Ingredients:

- 500g minced beef
- 2 tbsp gochujang
- 1 tbsp soy
- 2 tsp minced garlic
- 2 tsp minced ginger
- 2 tsp sugar
- 1 tbsp olive oil
- 1 chopped onion

Directions:

1. Mix all the ingredients in a large bowl, allow to rest for at least 30 minutes in the fridge
2. Divide the meat into four and form into patties
3. Place in the air fryer and cook at 180ºC for about 10 minutes
4. Serve in burger buns, if desired

Pork Schnitzel

Servings: 2
Cooking Time:xx
Ingredients:

- 3 pork steaks, cut into cubes
- Salt and pepper
- 175g flour
- 2 eggs
- 175g breadcrumbs

Directions:

1. Sprinkle the pork with salt and pepper
2. Coat in the flour then dip in the egg
3. Coat the pork in breadcrumbs
4. Place in the air fryer and cook at 175ºC for 20 minutes turning halfway
5. Serve with red cabbage

Beef Fried Rice

Servings: 2
Cooking Time:xx
Ingredients:

- 400g cooked rice
- 250g cooked beef strips
- 1 tbsp sesame oil
- 1 diced onion
- 1 egg
- 2 tsp garlic powder
- Salt and pepper
- 1 tbsp vegetable oil
- 250g frozen peas

Directions:

1. Preheat air fryer to 175ºC
2. Season the beef with salt, pepper and garlic powder, cook in a pan until about ¾ cooked
3. Mix the rice with peas carrots and vegetable oil, add the beef and mix
4. Add to the air fryer and cook for about 10 minutes
5. Add the egg and cook until the egg is done

Carne Asada Chips

Servings: 2
Cooking Time:xx

Ingredients:

- 500g sirloin steak
- 1 bag of frozen French fries
- 350g grated cheese
- 2 tbsp sour cream
- 2 tbsp guacamole
- 2 tbsp steak seasoning
- Salt and pepper to taste

Directions:

1. Preheat your oven to 260°C
2. Season the steak with the seasoning and a little salt and pepper
3. Place in the air fryer and cook for 4 minutes, before turning over and cooking for another 4 minutes
4. Remove and allow to rest
5. Add the French fries to the fryer and cook for 5 minutes, shaking regularly
6. Add the cheese
7. Cut the steak into pieces and add on top of the cheese
8. Cook for another 30 seconds, until the cheese is melted
9. Season

Traditional Pork Chops

Servings: 8
Cooking Time:xx

Ingredients:

- 8 pork chops
- 1 egg
- 100ml milk
- 300g bread crumbs
- 1 packet of dry ranch seasoning mix
- Salt and pepper to taste

Directions:

1. Preheat air fryer to 170°C
2. Beat the egg in a bowl, add the milk season with salt and pepper
3. In another bowl mix the bread crumbs and ranch dressing mix
4. Dip the pork into the egg then cover with breadcrumbs
5. Place in the air fryer and cook for 12 minutes turning half way

Fish & Seafood Recipes

Parmesan-coated Fish Fingers

Servings: 2
Cooking Time:xx
Ingredients:

- 350 g/12 oz. cod loins
- 1 tablespoon grated Parmesan
- 40 g/½ cup dried breadcrumbs (gluten-free if you wish, see page 9)
- 1 egg, beaten
- 2 tablespoons plain/all-purpose flour (gluten free if you wish)

Directions:

1. Slice the cod into 6 equal fish fingers/sticks.
2. Mix the Parmesan together with the breadcrumbs. Lay out three bowls: one with flour, one with beaten egg and the other with the Parmesan breadcrumbs. Dip each fish finger/stick first into the flour, then the egg and then the breadcrumbs until fully coated.
3. Preheat the air-fryer to 180°C/350°F.
4. Add the fish to the preheated air-fryer and air-fry for 6 minutes. Check the internal temperature of the fish has reached at least 75°C/167°F using a meat thermometer – if not, cook for another few minutes. Serve immediately.

Lemon Pepper Shrimp

Servings: 2
Cooking Time:xx
Ingredients:

- ½ tbsp olive oil
- The juice of 1 lemon
- ¼ tsp paprika
- 1 tsp lemon pepper
- ¼ tsp garlic powder
- 400g uncooked shrimp
- 1 sliced lemon

Directions:

1. Preheat air fryer to 200°C
2. Mix olive oil, lemon juice, paprika, lemon pepper and garlic powder. Add the shrimp and mix well
3. Place shrimp in the air fryer and cook for 6-8 minutes until pink and firm.
4. Serve with lemon slices

Shrimp With Yum Yum Sauce

Servings: 4
Cooking Time:xx
Ingredients:

- 400g peeled jumbo shrimp
- 1 tbsp soy sauce
- 1 tbsp garlic paste
- 1 tbsp ginger paste
- 4 tbsp mayo
- 2 tbsp ketchup
- 1 tbsp sugar
- 1 tsp paprika
- 1 tsp garlic powder

Directions:

1. Mix soy sauce, garlic paste and ginger paste in a bowl. Add the shrimp, allow to marinate for 15 minutes
2. In another bowl mix ketchup, mayo, sugar, paprika and the garlic powder to make the yum yum sauce.
3. Set the air fryer to 200°C, place shrimp in the basket and cook for 8-10 minutes

Store-cupboard Fishcakes

Servings: 3
Cooking Time:xx
Ingredients:

- 400 g/14 oz. cooked potato – either mashed potato or the insides of jacket potatoes (see page 124)
- 2 x 150–200-g/5½–7-oz. cans fish, such as tuna or salmon, drained
- 2 eggs
- ¾ teaspoon salt
- 1 teaspoon dried parsley
- ½ teaspoon freshly ground black pepper
- 1 tablespoon olive oil
- caper dressing (see page 79), to serve

Directions:

1. Mix the cooked potato, fish, eggs, salt, parsley and pepper together in a bowl, then divide into 6 equal portions and form into fishcakes. Drizzle the olive oil over both sides of each fishcake.
2. Preheat the air-fryer to 180ºC/350ºF.
3. Add the fishcakes to the preheated air-fryer and air-fry for 15 minutes, turning halfway through cooking. Serve with salad and tartare sauce or Caper Dressing.

Cajun Shrimp Boil

Servings: 6
Cooking Time:xx
Ingredients:

- 300g cooked shrimp
- 14 slices of smoked sausage
- 5 par boiled potatoes, cut into halves
- 4 mini corn on the cobs, quartered
- 1 diced onion
- 3 tbsp old bay seasoning
- Olive oil spray

Directions:

1. Combine all the ingredients in a bowl and mix well
2. Line the air fryer with foil
3. Place half the mix into the air fryer and cook at 200ºC for about 6 minutes, mix the ingredients and cook for a further 6 minutes.
4. Repeat for the second batch

Maine Seafood

Servings: 2
Cooking Time:xx
Ingredients:

- 500g flour
- 400g breadcrumbs
- 300g steamer clams
- 3 eggs
- 3 tbsp water

Directions:

1. Soak the clams for 3 hours, drain and rinse
2. Bring 1 inch of water to boil, add the clams and cover with a lid, steam for about 7 minutes until the clams open.
3. Remove the clams from the shell and set aside
4. Put the eggs in a bowl and mix with the water
5. Dip the clams in the flour, then the egg and then coat in breadcrumbs
6. Heat the air fryer to 180ºC and cook for about 7 minutes

Gluten Free Honey And Garlic Shrimp

Servings: 2
Cooking Time:xx

Ingredients:

- 500g fresh shrimp
- 5 tbsp honey
- 2 tbsp gluten free soy sauce
- 2 tbsp tomato ketchup
- 250g frozen stir fry vegetables
- 1 crushed garlic clove
- 1 tsp fresh ginger
- 2 tbsp cornstarch

Directions:

1. Simmer the honey, soy sauce, garlic, tomato ketchup and ginger in a saucepan
2. Add the cornstarch and whisk until sauce thickens
3. Coat the shrimp with the sauce
4. Line the air fryer with foil and add the shrimp and vegetables
5. Cook at 180ºC for 10 minutes

Cod In Parma Ham

Servings: 2
Cooking Time:xx

Ingredients:

- 2 x 175–190-g/6–7-oz. cod fillets, skin removed
- 6 slices Parma ham or prosciutto
- 16 cherry tomatoes
- 60 g/2 oz. rocket/arugula
- DRESSING
- 1 tablespoon olive oil
- 1½ teaspoons balsamic vinegar
- garlic salt, to taste
- freshly ground black pepper, to taste

Directions:

1. Preheat the air-fryer to 180ºC/350ºF.
2. Wrap each piece of cod snugly in 3 ham slices. Add the ham-wrapped cod fillets and the tomatoes to the preheated air-fryer and air-fry for 6 minutes, turning the cod halfway through cooking. Check the internal temperature of the fish has reached at least 60ºC/140ºF using a meat thermometer – if not, cook for another minute.
3. Meanwhile, make the dressing by combining all the ingredients in a jar and shaking well.
4. Serve the cod and tomatoes on a bed of rocket/arugula with the dressing poured over.

Pesto Salmon

Servings: 4
Cooking Time:xx

Ingredients:

- 4 x 150–175-g/5½–6-oz. salmon fillets
- lemon wedges, to serve
- PESTO
- 50 g/scant ½ cup toasted pine nuts
- 50 g/2 oz. fresh basil
- 50 g/⅔ cup grated Parmesan or Pecorino
- 100 ml/7 tablespoons olive oil

Directions:

1. To make the pesto, blitz the pine nuts, basil and Parmesan to a paste in a food processor. Pour in the olive oil and process again.
2. Preheat the air-fryer to 160ºC/325ºF.
3. Top each salmon fillet with 2 tablespoons of the pesto. Add the salmon fillets to the preheated air-fryer and air-fry for 9 minutes. Check the internal temperature of the fish has reached at least 63ºC/145ºF using a meat thermometer – if not, cook for another few minutes.

Mahi Fish Tacos

Servings: 4
Cooking Time:xx

Ingredients:

- 400g fresh mahi
- 8 small corn tortillas
- 2 tsp cajun seasoning
- 5 tbsp sour cream
- 2 tbsp mayonnaise
- 2 tbsp scotch bonnet pepper sauce (use 1 tbsp if you don't like your food too spicy)
- 1 tbsp sriracha sauce
- 2 tbsp lime juice
- Salt and pepper to taste
- 1 tbsp vegetable oil

Directions:

1. Clean the mahi. Cut into half inch slices and season with salt
2. Mix quarter parts cayenne pepper and black pepper with cajun seasoning. Sprinkle onto fish
3. Brush pepper sauce on both sides of the fish
4. Set the air fryer to 180ºC and cook for about 10 minutes or until golden brown
5. Whilst the fish cooks make the chipotle lime cream. Mix the mayo, sour cream, lime juice sriracha and cayenne pepper
6. Assemble tacos and enjoy

Salmon Patties

Servings: 4
Cooking Time:xx

Ingredients:

- 400g salmon
- 1 egg
- 1 diced onion
- 200g breadcrumbs
- 1 tsp dill weed

Directions:

1. Remove all bones and skin from the salmon
2. Mix egg, onion, dill weed and bread crumbs with the salmon
3. Shape mixture into patties and place into the air fryer
4. Set air fryer to 180ºC
5. Cook for 5 minutes then turn them over and cook for a further 5 minutes until golden brown

Fish Sticks With Tartar Sauce Batter

Servings: 4
Cooking Time:xx

Ingredients:

- 6 tbsp mayonnaise
- 2 tbsp dill pickle
- 1 tsp seafood seasoning
- 400g cod fillets, cut into sticks
- 300g panko breadcrumbs

Directions:

1. Combine the mayonnaise, seafood seasoning and dill pickle in a large bowl.
2. Add the cod sticks and coat well
3. Preheat air fryer to 200ºC
4. Coat the fish sticks in the breadcrumbs
5. Place in the air fryer and cook for 12 minutes

Mushrooms Stuffed With Crab

Servings: 2
Cooking Time:xx

Ingredients:

- 500g large mushrooms
- 2 tsp salt
- Half a diced red onion
- 2 diced celery sticks
- 300g lump crab
- 35g seasoned breadcrumbs
- 1 egg
- 1 tsp oregano
- 1 tsp hot sauce
- 50g grated Parmesan cheese

Directions:

1. Preheat to 260ºC
2. Take a baking sheet and arrange the mushrooms top down
3. Spray with a little cooking oil
4. Take a bowl and combine the onions, celery, breadcrumbs, egg, crab and half the cheese, oregano and hot sauce
5. Fill each mushroom with the mixture and make sure it's heaped over the top
6. Cover with the rest of the cheese
7. Place in the air fryer for 18 minutes

Crispy Nacho Prawns

Servings: 6
Cooking Time:xx

Ingredients:

- 1 egg
- 18 large prawns
- 1 bag of nacho cheese flavoured corn chips, crushed

Directions:

1. Wash the prawns and pat dry
2. Place the chips into a bowl
3. In another bowl, whisk the egg
4. Dip the prawns into the egg and then the nachos
5. Preheat the air fryer to 180°C
6. Cook for 8 minutes

Salt & Pepper Calamari

Servings: 2
Cooking Time:xx

Ingredients:

- 500g squid rings
- 500g panko breadcrumbs
- 250g plain flour
- 2 tbsp pepper
- 2 tbsp salt
- 200ml buttermilk
- 1 egg

Directions:

1. Take a medium bowl and combine the buttermilk and egg, stirring well
2. Take another bowl and combine the salt, pepper, flour, and panko breadcrumbs, combining again
3. Dip the quid into the buttermilk first and then the breadcrumbs, coating evenly
4. Place in the air fryer basket
5. Cook at 150°C for 12 minutes, until golden

Fish In Parchment Paper

Servings: 2
Cooking Time:xx

Ingredients:

- 250g cod fillets
- 1 chopped carrot
- 1 chopped fennel
- 1 tbsp oil
- 1 thinly sliced red pepper
- ½ tsp tarragon
- 1 tbsp lemon juice
- 1 tbsp salt
- ½ tsp ground pepper

Directions:

1. In a bowl, mix the tarragon and ½ tsp salt add the vegetables and mix well
2. Cut two large squares of parchment paper
3. Spray the cod with oil and cover both sides with salt and pepper
4. Place the cod in the parchment paper and add the vegetables
5. Fold over the paper to hold the fish and vegetables
6. Place in the air fryer and cook at 170°C for 15 minutes

Fish In Foil

Servings: 2
Cooking Time:xx

Ingredients:

- 1 tablespoon avocado oil or olive oil, plus extra for greasing
- 1 tablespoon soy sauce (or tamari)
- 1½ teaspoons freshly grated garlic
- 1½ teaspoons freshly grated ginger
- 1 small red chilli/chile, finely chopped
- 2 skinless, boneless white fish fillets (about 350 g/12 oz. total weight)

Directions:

1. Mix the oil, soy sauce, garlic, ginger and chilli/chile together. Brush a little oil onto two pieces of foil, then lay the fish in the centre of the foil. Spoon the topping mixture over the fish. Wrap the foil around the fish to make a parcel, with a gap above the fish but shallow enough to fit in your air-fryer basket.
2. Preheat the air-fryer to 180°C/350°F.
3. Add the foil parcels to the preheated air-fryer and air-fry for 7–10 minutes, depending on the thickness of your fillets. The fish should just flake when a fork is inserted. Serve immediately.

Garlic-parsley Prawns

Servings: 2
Cooking Time:xx

Ingredients:

- 300 g/10½ oz. raw king prawns/jumbo shrimp (without shell)
- 40 g/3 tablespoons garlic butter, softened (see page 72)
- 2 tablespoons freshly chopped flat-leaf parsley

Directions:

1. Thread the prawns/shrimp onto 6 metal skewers that will fit your air-fryer. Mix together the softened garlic butter and parsley and brush evenly onto the prawn skewers.
2. Preheat the air-fryer to 180°C/350°F.
3. Place the skewers on an air-fryer liner or a piece of pierced parchment paper. Add the skewers to the preheated air-fryer and air-fry for 2 minutes, then turn the skewers over and cook for a further 2 minutes. Check the internal temperature of the prawns has reached at least 50°C/120°F using a meat thermometer – if not, cook for another few minutes and serve.

Honey Sriracha Salmon

Servings: 2
Cooking Time:xx

Ingredients:

- 25g sriracha
- 25g honey
- 500g salmon fillets
- 1 tbsp soy sauce

Directions:

1. Mix the honey, soy sauce and sriracha, keep half the mix to one side for dipping
2. Place the salmon in the sauce skin side up and marinade for 30 minutes
3. Spray air fryer basket with cooking spray
4. Heat the air fryer to 200°C
5. Place salmon in the air fryer skin side down and cook for 12 minutes

Beer Battered Fish Tacos

Servings: 2
Cooking Time:xx

Ingredients:

- 300g cod fillets
- 2 eggs
- 1 can of Mexican beer
- 300g cornstarch
- 300g flour
- 2 soft corn tortillas
- ½ tsp chilli powder
- 1 tbsp cumin
- Salt and pepper to taste

Directions:

1. Whisk together the eggs and beer
2. In a separate bowl whisk together cornstarch, chilli powder, flour, cumin and salt and pepper
3. Coat the fish in the egg mixture then coat in flour mixture
4. Spray the air fryer with non stick spray and add the fish
5. Set your fryer to 170°C and cook for 15 minutes
6. Place the fish in a corn tortilla

Vegetarian & Vegan Recipes

Tofu Bowls

Servings: 4
Cooking Time:xx
Ingredients:

- 1 block of tofu, cut into cubes
- 40ml soy sauce
- 2 tbsp sesame oil
- 1 tsp garlic powder
- 1 chopped onion
- 2 tbsp Tahini dressing
- 3 bunches baby bok choy, chopped
- 300g quinoa
- 1 medium cucumber, sliced
- 1 cup shredded carrot
- 1 avocado, sliced

Directions:

1. Mix the soy sauce, 1 tbsp sesame oil and garlic powder in a bowl. Add the tofu marinade for 10 minutes
2. Place in the air fryer and cook at 200ºC for 20 minutes turning halfway
3. Heat the remaining sesame oil in a pan and cook the onions for about 4 minutes
4. Add the bok choy and cook for another 4 minutes
5. Divide the quinoa between your bowls add bok choy, carrot, cucumber and avocado. Top with the tofu and drizzle with Tahini

Pakoras

Servings: 8
Cooking Time:xx
Ingredients:

- 200g chopped cauliflower
- 100g diced pepper
- 250g chickpea flour
- 30ml water
- ½ tsp cumin
- Cooking spray
- 1 onion, diced
- 1 tsp salt
- 1 garlic clove, minced
- 1 tsp curry powder
- 1 tsp coriander
- ½ tsp cayenne

Directions:

1. Preheat air fryer to 175ºC
2. Place all ingredients in a bowl and mix well
3. Spray cooking basket with oil
4. Spoon 2 tbsp of mix into the basket and flatten, continue until the basket is full
5. Cook for 8 minutes, turn then cook for a further 8 minutes

Onion Dumplings

Servings: 2
Cooking Time:xx

Ingredients:

- 14 frozen dumplings (pierogies)
- 1 onion
- 1 tbsp olive oil
- 1 tsp sugar

Directions:

1. Take a large saucepan and fill with water, bringing to the boil
2. Cook the dumplings for 5 minutes, remove and drain
3. Slice the onion into long pieces
4. Oil the air fryer basket and preheat to 220ºC
5. Cook the onion for 12 minutes, stirring often. After 5 minutes, add the sugar and combine
6. Remove the onions and place to one side
7. Add the dumplings to the air fryer and cook for 4 minutes
8. Turn the temperature up to 270ºC and cook for another 3 minutes
9. Mix the dumplings with the onions before serving

Courgette Meatballs

Servings: 4
Cooking Time:xx

Ingredients:

- 400g oats
- 40g feta, crumbled
- 1 beaten egg
- Salt and pepper
- 150g courgette
- 1 tsp lemon rind
- 6 basil leaves, thinly sliced
- 1 tsp dill
- 1 tsp oregano

Directions:

1. Preheat the air fryer to 200ºC
2. Grate the courgette into a bowl, squeeze any access water out
3. Add all the remaining ingredients apart from the oats and mix well
4. Blend the oats until they resemble breadcrumbs
5. Add the oats into the other mix and stir well
6. Form into balls and place in the air fryer cook for 10 minutes

Spicy Spanish Potatoes

Servings: 2
Cooking Time:xx

Ingredients:

- 4 large potatoes
- 1 tbsp olive oil
- 2 tsp paprika
- 2 tsp dried garlic
- 1 tsp barbacoa seasoning
- Salt and pepper

Directions:

1. Chop the potatoes into wedges
2. Place them in a bowl with olive oil and seasoning, mix well
3. Add to the air fryer and cook at 160ºC for 20 minutes
4. Shake, increase heat to 200ºC and cook for another 3 minutes

Spinach And Feta Croissants

Servings:4
Cooking Time:10 Minutes

Ingredients:

- 4 pre-made croissants
- 100 g / 7 oz feta cheese, crumbled
- 1 tsp dried chives
- 1 tsp garlic powder
- 50 g / 3.5 oz fresh spinach, chopped

Directions:

1. Preheat the air fryer to 180 °C / 350 °F. Remove the mesh basket from the air fryer machine and line with parchment paper.
2. Cut the croissants in half and lay each half out on the lined mesh basket.
3. In a bowl, combine the crumbled feta cheese, dried chives, garlic powder, and chopped spinach until they form a consistent mixture.
4. Spoon some of the mixture one half of the four croissants and cover with the second half of the croissants to seal in the filling.
5. Carefully slide the croissants in the mesh basket into the air fryer machine, close the lid, and cook for 10 minutes until the pastry is crispy and the feta cheese has melted.

Vegan Meatballs

Servings:4
Cooking Time:15 Minutes

Ingredients:

- 2 tbsp olive oil
- 2 tbsp soy sauce
- 1 onion, finely sliced
- 1 large carrot, peeled and grated
- 1 x 400 g / 14 oz can chickpeas, drained and rinsed
- 50 g / 1.8 oz plain flour
- 50 g / 1.8 oz rolled oats
- 2 tbsp roasted cashews, chopped
- 1 tsp garlic powder
- ½ tsp cumin

Directions:

1. Preheat the air fryer to 175 °C / 350 °F and line the air fryer with parchment paper or grease it with olive oil.
2. In a large mixing bowl, combine the olive oil and soy sauce. Add the onion slices and grated carrot and toss to coat in the sauce.
3. Place the vegetables in the air fryer and cook for 5 minutes until slightly soft.
4. Meanwhile, place the chickpeas, plain flour, rolled oats, and roasted cashews in a blender, and mix until well combined.
5. Remove the mixture from the blender and stir in the garlic powder and cumin. Add the onions and carrots to the bowl and mix well.
6. Scoop the mixture into small meatballs and place them into the air fryer. Increase the temperature on the machine up to 190 °C / 370 °F and cook the meatballs for 10-12 minutes until golden and crispy.

Miso Mushrooms On Sourdough Toast

Servings: 1
Cooking Time:xx

Ingredients:

- 1 teaspoon miso paste
- 1 teaspoon oil, such as avocado or coconut (melted)
- 1 teaspoon soy sauce
- 80 g/3 oz. chestnut mushrooms, sliced 5 mm/½ in. thick
- 1 large slice sourdough bread
- 2 teaspoons butter or plant-based spread
- a little freshly chopped flat-leaf parsley, to serve

Directions:

1. Preheat the air-fryer to 200ºC/400ºF.
2. In a small bowl or ramekin mix together the miso paste, oil and soy sauce.
3. Place the mushrooms in a small shallow gratin dish that fits inside your air-fryer. Add the sauce to the mushrooms and mix together. Place the gratin dish in the preheated air-fryer and air-fry for 6–7 minutes, stirring once during cooking.
4. With 4 minutes left to cook, add the bread to the air-fryer and turn over at 2 minutes whilst giving the mushrooms a final stir.
5. Once cooked, butter the toast and serve the mushrooms on top, scattered with chopped parsley.

Tempura Veggies

Servings: 4
Cooking Time:xx

Ingredients:

- 150g flour
- ½ tsp salt
- ½ tsp pepper
- 2 eggs
- 2 tbsp cup water
- 100g avocado wedges
- 100g courgette slices
- 100g panko breadcrumbs
- 2 tsp oil
- 100g green beans
- 100g asparagus spears
- 100g red onion rings
- 100g pepper rings

Directions:

1. Mix together flour, salt and pepper. In another bowl mix eggs and water
2. Stir together panko crumbs and oil in a separate bowl
3. Dip vegetables in the flour mix, then egg and then the bread crumbs
4. Preheat the air fryer to 200°C
5. Place in the air fryer and cook for about 10 minutes until golden brown

Spanakopita Bites

Servings: 4
Cooking Time:xx

Ingredients:

- 300g baby spinach
- 2 tbsp water
- 100g cottage cheese
- 50g feta cheese
- 2 tbsp grated parmesan
- 1 tbsp olive oil
- 4 sheets of filo pastry
- 1 large egg white
- 1 tsp lemon zest
- 1 tsp oregano
- ¼ tsp salt
- ¼ tsp pepper
- ⅛ tsp cayenne

Directions:

1. Place spinach in water and cook for about 5 minutes, drain
2. Mix all ingredients together
3. Place a sheet of pastry down and brush with oil, place another on the top and do the same, continue until all four on top of each other
4. Ut the pastry into 8 strips then cut each strip in half across the middle
5. Add 1 tbsp of mix to each piece of pastry
6. Fold one corner over the mix to create a triangle, fold over the other corner to seal
7. Place in the air fryer and cook at 190°C for about 12 minutes until golden brown

Broccoli Cheese

Servings: 2
Cooking Time:xx

Ingredients:

- 250g broccoli
- Cooking spray
- 10 tbsp evaporated milk
- 300g Mexican cheese
- 4 tsp Amarillo paste
- 6 saltine crackers

Directions:

1. Heat the air fryer to 190ºC
2. Place the broccoli in the air fryer spray with cooking oil and cook for about 6 minutes
3. Place the remaining ingredients in a blender and process until smooth
4. Place in a bowl and microwave for 30 seconds
5. Pour over the broccoli and serve

Paneer Tikka

Servings: 2
Cooking Time:xx

Ingredients:

- 200ml yogurt
- 1 tsp ginger garlic paste
- 1 tsp red chilli powder
- 1 tsp garam masala
- 1 tsp turmeric powder
- 1 tbsp dried fenugreek leaves
- The juice of 1 lemon
- 2 tbsp chopped coriander
- 1 tbsp olive oil
- 250g paneer cheese, cut into cubes
- 1 green pepper, chopped
- 1 red pepper, chopped
- 1 yellow pepper, chopped
- 1 chopped onion

Directions:

1. Take a mixing bowl and add the yogurt, garlic paste, red chilli powder, garam masala, turmeric powder, lemon juice, fenugreek and chopped coriander, combining well
2. Place the marinade to one side
3. Add the cubed cheese to the marinade and toss to coat well
4. Leave to marinade for 2 hours
5. Take 8 skewers and alternate the cheese with the peppers and onions
6. Drizzle a little oil over the top
7. Arrange in the air fryer and cook at 220ºC for 3 minutes
8. Turn and cook for another 3 minutes

Bbq Soy Curls

Servings: 2
Cooking Time:xx
Ingredients:

- 250ml warm water
- 1 tsp vegetable bouillon
- 200g soy curls
- 40g BBQ sauce
- 1 tsp oil

Directions:

1. Soak the soy curls in water and bouillon for 10 minutes
2. Place the soy curls in another bowl and shred
3. Heat the air fryer to 200°C
4. Cook for 3 minutes
5. Remove from the air fryer and coat in bbq sauce
6. Return to the air fryer and cook for 5 minutes shaking halfway through

Vegan Fried Ravioli

Servings: 4
Cooking Time:xx
Ingredients:

- 100g panko breadcrumbs
- 2 tsp yeast
- 1 tsp basil
- 1 tsp oregano
- 1 tsp garlic powder
- Pinch salt and pepper
- 50ml liquid from can of chickpeas
- 150g vegan ravioli
- Cooking spray
- 50g marinara for dipping

Directions:

1. Combine the breadcrumbs, yeast, basil, oregano, garlic powder and salt and pepper
2. Put the liquid from the chickpeas in a bowl
3. Dip the ravioli in the liquid then dip into the breadcrumb mix
4. Heat the air fryer to 190°C
5. Place the ravioli in the air fryer and cook for about 6 minutes until crispy

Goat's Cheese Tartlets

Servings: 2
Cooking Time:xx
Ingredients:

- 1 readymade sheet of puff pastry, 35 x 23 cm/14 x 9 in. (gluten-free if you wish)
- 4 tablespoons pesto (jarred or see page 80)
- 4 roasted baby (bell) peppers (see page 120)
- 4 tablespoons soft goat's cheese
- 2 teaspoons milk (plant-based if you wish)

Directions:

1. Cut the pastry sheet in half along the long edge, to make two smaller rectangles. Fold in the edges of each pastry rectangle to form a crust. Using a fork, prick a few holes in the base of the pastry. Brush half the pesto onto each rectangle, top with the peppers and goat's cheese. Brush the pastry crust with milk.
2. Preheat the air-fryer to 180°C/350°F.
3. Place one tartlet on an air-fryer liner or a piece of pierced parchment paper in the preheated air-fryer and air-fry for 6 minutes (you'll need to cook them one at a time). Repeat with the second tartlet.

Mini Quiche

Servings: 2
Cooking Time:xx

Ingredients:

- 100g raw cashews
- 3 tbsp milk
- ½ tsp hot sauce
- 1 tsp white miso paste
- 1 tsp mustard
- 300g tofu
- 100g bacon pieces
- 1 chopped red pepper
- 1 chopped onion
- 6 tbsp yeast
- ½ tsp onion powder
- ½ tsp paprika
- ½ tsp cumin
- ½ tsp chilli powder
- ½ tsp black pepper
- ⅛ tsp turmeric
- ½ tsp canola oil
- 50g curly kale

Directions:

1. Heat the oil in a pan, add the bacon pepper, onion and curly kale and cook for about 3 minutes
2. Place all the other ingredients into a blender and blend until smooth
3. Add to a bowl with the bacon, pepper, onion and curly kale and mix well
4. Fill silicone muffin cups with the mix
5. Place in the air fryer and cook at 165°C for 15 minutes

Quinoa-stuffed Romano Peppers

Servings: 2
Cooking Time:xx

Ingredients:

- 1 tablespoon olive oil
- 1 onion, diced
- 1 garlic clove, chopped
- 100 g/⅔ cup uncooked quinoa
- 1½ tablespoons fajita seasoning
- 140 g/1 cup canned sweetcorn/corn kernels (drained weight)
- 3 romano peppers, sliced lengthways, seeds removed but stalk left intact
- 60 g/⅔ cup grated mature Cheddar

Directions:

1. Heat the oil in a saucepan. Add the onion and garlic and sauté for 5 minutes, until soft. Add the quinoa, fajita seasoning and 250 ml/1 cup water. Bring to a simmer, then cover with a lid and simmer for 15 minutes or until the quinoa is cooked and the water absorbed. Stir in the sweetcorn/corn kernels. Stuff each pepper half with the quinoa mixture, then top with grated cheese.
2. Preheat the air-fryer to 180°C/350°F.
3. Place the peppers on an air-fryer liner or a piece of pierced parchment paper, place in the preheated air-fryer and air-fry for 12–14 minutes, depending how 'chargrilled' you like your peppers.

Saganaki

Servings: 2
Cooking Time:xx

Ingredients:

- 200 g/7 oz. kefalotyri or manouri cheese, sliced into wedges 1 cm/½ in. thick
- 2 tablespoons plain/all-purpose flour
- olive oil, for drizzling

Directions:

1. Preheat the air-fryer to 200ºC/400ºF.
2. Dip each wedge of cheese in the flour, then tap off any excess. Drizzle olive oil onto both sides of the cheese slices
3. Add the cheese to the preheated air-fryer and air-fry for 3 minutes. Remove from the air-fryer and serve.

Bagel Pizza

Servings: 1
Cooking Time:xx

Ingredients:

- 1 bagel
- 2 tbsp marinara sauce
- 6 slices vegan pepperoni
- 2 tbsp mozzarella
- Pinch of basil

Directions:

1. Heat the air fryer to 180ºC
2. Cut the bagel in half and toast for 2 minutes in the air fryer
3. Remove from the air fryer and top with marinara sauce, pepperoni and mozzarella
4. Return to the air fryer and cook for 4-5 minutes
5. Sprinkle with basil to serve

Veggie Lasagne

Servings: 1
Cooking Time:xx

Ingredients:

- 2 lasagne sheets
- Pinch of salt
- 100g pasta sauce
- 50g ricotta
- 60g chopped basil
- 40g chopped spinach
- 3 tbsp grated courgette

Directions:

1. Break the lasagne sheets in half, bring a pan of water to boil
2. Cook the lasagne sheets for about 8 minutes, drain and pat dry
3. Add 2 tbsp of pasta sauce to a mini loaf tin
4. Add a lasagne sheet, top with ricotta, basil and spinach, then add courgette
5. Place another lasagne sheet on top
6. Add a couple of tbsp pasta sauce, basil, spinach and courgette
7. Add the last lasagne sheet, top with pasta sauce and ricotta
8. Cover with foil and place in the air fryer
9. Cook at 180ºC for 10 mins, remove foil and cook for another 3 minutes

Side Dishes Recipes

Mediterranean Vegetables

Servings: 1–2
Cooking Time:xx
Ingredients:

- 1 courgette/zucchini, thickly sliced
- 1 (bell) pepper, deseeded and chopped into large chunks
- 1 red onion, sliced into wedges
- 12 cherry tomatoes
- 1 tablespoon olive oil
- ½ teaspoon salt
- ½ teaspoon freshly ground black pepper
- 2 rosemary twigs
- mozzarella, fresh pesto (see page 80) and basil leaves, to serve

Directions:

1. Preheat the air-fryer to 180°C/350°F.
2. Toss the prepared vegetables in the oil and seasoning. Add the vegetables and the rosemary to the preheated air-fryer and air-fry for 12–14 minutes, depending on how 'chargrilled' you like them.
3. Remove and serve topped with fresh mozzarella and pesto and scattered with basil leaves.

Sweet & Spicy Baby Peppers

Servings: 2
Cooking Time:xx
Ingredients:

- 200 g/7 oz. piccarella (baby) peppers, deseeded and quartered lengthways
- 1 teaspoon olive oil
- ½ teaspoon chilli/chili paste
- ¼ teaspoon runny honey
- salt and freshly ground black pepper

Directions:

1. Preheat the air-fryer to 180°C/350°F.
2. Toss the peppers in the oil, chilli/chili paste and honey, then add salt and pepper to taste.
3. Place in the preheated air-fryer and air-fry for 6–8 minutes, depending on how 'chargrilled' you like them, turning them over halfway through.

Cheesy Garlic Asparagus

Servings: 4
Cooking Time:xx
Ingredients:

- 1 tsp olive oil
- 500g asparagus
- 1 tsp garlic salt
- 1 tbsp grated parmesan cheese
- Salt and pepper for seasoning

Directions:

1. Preheat the air fryer to 270°C
2. Clean the asparagus and cut off the bottom 1"
3. Pat dry and place in the air fryer, covering with the oil
4. Sprinkle the parmesan and garlic salt on top, seasoning to your liking
5. Cook for between 7 and 10 minutes
6. Add a little extra parmesan over the top before serving

Bbq Beetroot Crisps

Servings:4
Cooking Time:5 Minutes

Ingredients:

- 400 g / 14 oz beetroot, sliced
- 2 tbsp olive oil
- 1 tbsp BBQ seasoning
- ½ tsp black pepper

Directions:

1. Preheat the air fryer to 180 °C / 350 °F and line the bottom of the basket with parchment paper.
2. Place the beetroot slices in a large bowl. Add the olive oil, BBQ seasoning, and black pepper, and toss to coat the beetroot slices on both sides.
3. Place the beetroot slices in the air fryer and cook for 5 minutes until hot and crispy.

Courgette Gratin

Servings: 2
Cooking Time:xx

Ingredients:

- 2 courgette
- 1 tbsp chopped parsley
- 2 tbsp breadcrumbs
- 4 tbsp grated parmesan
- 1 tbsp vegetable oil
- Salt and pepper to taste

Directions:

1. Heat the air fryer to 180ºC
2. Cut each courgette in half length ways then slice
3. Mix the remaining ingredients together
4. Place the courgette in the air fryer and top with the breadcrumb mix
5. Cook for about 15 minutes until golden brown

Whole Sweet Potatoes

Servings: 4 As A Side Or Snack
Cooking Time:xx

Ingredients:

- 4 medium sweet potatoes
- 1 tablespoon olive oil
- 1 teaspoon salt
- toppings of your choice

Directions:

1. Preheat the air-fryer to 200ºC/400ºF.
2. Wash and remove any imperfections from the skin of the sweet potatoes, then rub the potatoes with the olive oil and salt.
3. Add the sweet potatoes to the preheated air-fryer and air-fry for up to 40 minutes (the cooking time depends on the size of the potatoes). Remove as soon as they are soft when pierced. Slice open and serve with your choice of toppings.
4. VARIATION: WHOLE JACKET POTATOES
5. Regular baking potatoes can be air-fried in the same way, but will require a cooking time of 45–60 minutes, depending on their size.

Ranch-style Potatoes

Servings: 2
Cooking Time:xx

Ingredients:

- 300g baby potatoes, washed
- 1 tbsp olive oil
- 3 tbsp dry ranch seasoning

Directions:

1. Preheat the air fryer to 220ºC
2. Cut the potatoes in half
3. Take a mixing bowl and combine the olive oil with the ranch seasoning
4. Add the potatoes to the bowl and toss to coat
5. Cook for 15 minutes, shaking halfway through

Potato Wedges

Servings: 4
Cooking Time:xx

Ingredients:

- 2 potatoes, cut into wedges
- 1 ½ tbsp olive oil
- ½ tsp paprika
- ⅛ tsp ground black pepper
- ½ tsp parsley flakes
- ½ tsp chilli powder
- ½ tsp sea salt

Directions:

1. Preheat the air fryer to 200ºC
2. Add all ingredients to a bowl and combine well
3. Place the wedges into the air fryer and cook for 10 minutes
4. Turn and cook for a further 8 minutes until golden brown

Cauliflower With Hot Sauce And Blue Cheese Sauce

Servings:2
Cooking Time:15 Minutes

Ingredients:

- For the cauliflower:
- 1 cauliflower, broken into florets
- 4 tbsp hot sauce
- 2 tbsp olive oil
- 1 tsp garlic powder
- ½ tsp salt
- ½ tsp black pepper
- 1 tbsp plain flour
- 1 tbsp corn starch
- For the blue cheese sauce:
- 50 g / 1.8 oz blue cheese, crumbled
- 2 tbsp sour cream
- 2 tbsp mayonnaise
- ½ tsp salt
- ½ tsp black pepper

Directions:

1. Preheat the air fryer to 180 °C / 350 °F and line the bottom of the basket with parchment paper.
2. In a bowl, combine the hot sauce, olive oil, garlic powder, salt, and black pepper until it forms a consistent mixture. Add the cauliflower to the bowl and coat in the sauce.
3. Stir in the plain flour and corn starch until well combined.
4. Transfer the cauliflower to the lined basket in the air fryer, close the lid, and cook for 12-15 minutes until the cauliflower has softened and is golden in colour.
5. Meanwhile, make the blue cheese sauce by combining all of the ingredients. When the cauliflower is ready, remove it from the air fryer and serve with the blue cheese sauce on the side.

Roasted Brussels Sprouts

Servings: 3

Cooking Time:xx

Ingredients:

- 300 g/10½ oz. Brussels sprouts, trimmed and halved
- 1 tablespoon olive oil
- ½ teaspoon salt
- ¼ teaspoon freshly ground black pepper

Directions:

1. Preheat the air-fryer to 160ºC/325ºF.
2. Toss the Brussels sprout halves in the oil and the seasoning. Add these to the preheated air-fryer and air-fry for 15 minutes, then increase the temperature of the air-fryer to 180ºC/350ºF and cook for a further 5 minutes until the sprouts are really crispy on the outside and cooked through.

Sweet And Sticky Parsnips And Carrots

Servings:2

Cooking Time:15 Minutes

Ingredients:

- 4 large carrots, peeled and chopped into long chunks
- 4 large parsnips, peeled and chopped into long chunks
- 1 tbsp olive oil
- 2 tbsp honey
- 1 tsp dried mixed herbs

Directions:

1. Preheat the air fryer to 150 °C / 300 °F and line the bottom of the basket with parchment paper.
2. Place the chopped carrots and parsnips in a large bowl and drizzle over the olive oil and honey. Sprinkle in some black pepper to taste and toss well to fully coat the vegetables.
3. Transfer the coated vegetables into the air fryer basket and shut the lid. Cook for 20 minutes until the carrots and parsnips and cooked and crispy.
4. Serve as a side with your dinner.

Potato Hay

Servings: 4

Cooking Time:xx

Ingredients:

- 2 potatoes
- 1 tbsp oil
- Salt and pepper to taste

Directions:

1. Cut the potatoes into spirals
2. Soak in a bowl of water for 20 minutes, drain and pat dry
3. Add oil, salt and pepper and mix well to coat
4. Preheat air fryer to 180ºC
5. Add potatoes to air fryer and cook for 5 minutes, toss then cook for another 12 until golden brown

Courgette Chips

Servings: 4
Cooking Time:xx

Ingredients:

- 250g panko bread crumbs
- 100g grated parmesan
- 1 medium courgette, thinly sliced
- 1 egg beaten

Directions:

1. Preheat the air fryer to 175°C
2. Combine the breadcrumbs and parmesan
3. Dip the courgette into the egg then coat in bread crumbs
4. Spray with cooking spray and cook in the air fryer for 10 minutes
5. Turnover with tongs and cook for a further 2 minutes

Asparagus Fries

Servings: 2
Cooking Time:xx

Ingredients:

- 1 egg
- 1 tsp honey
- 100g panko bread crumbs
- Pinch of cayenne pepper
- 100g grated parmesan
- 12 asparagus spears
- 75g mustard
- 75g Greek yogurt

Directions:

1. Preheat air fryer to 200°C
2. Combine egg and honey in a bowl, mix panko crumbs and parmesan on a plate
3. Coat each asparagus in egg then in the bread crumbs
4. Place in the air fryer and cook for about 6 mins
5. Mix the remaining ingredients in a bowl and serve as a dipping sauce

Air Fryer Eggy Bread

Servings:2
Cooking Time:5-7 Minutes

Ingredients:

- 4 slices white bread
- 4 eggs, beaten
- 1 tsp black pepper
- 1 tsp dried chives

Directions:

1. Preheat your air fryer to 150 °C / 300 °F and line the bottom of the basket with parchment paper.
2. Whisk the eggs in a large mixing bowl and soak each slice of bread until fully coated.
3. Transfer the eggy bread to the preheated air fryer and cook for 5-7 minutes until the eggs are set and the bread is crispy.
4. Serve hot with a sprinkle of black pepper and chives on top.

Potato Wedges With Rosemary

Servings: 2
Cooking Time:xx

Ingredients:

- 2 potatoes, sliced into wedges
- 1 tbsp olive oil
- 2 tsp seasoned salt
- 2 tbsp chopped rosemary

Directions:

1. Preheat air fryer to 190ºC
2. Drizzle potatoes with oil, mix in salt and rosemary
3. Place in the air fryer and cook for 20 minutes turning halfway

Ricotta Stuffed Aubergine

Servings: 2
Cooking Time:xx

Ingredients:

- 1 aubergine
- 150g ricotta cheese
- 75g Parmesan cheese, plus an extra 75g for the breading
- 1 tsp garlic powder
- 3 tbsp parsley
- 1 egg, plus an extra 2 eggs for the breading
- 300g pork rind crumbs
- 2 tsp Italian seasoning

Directions:

1. Cut the aubergine into rounds, about 1/2" in thickness
2. Line a baking sheet with parchment and arrange the rounds on top, sprinkling with salt
3. Place another sheet of parchment on top and place something heavy on top to get rid of excess water
4. Leave for 30 minutes
5. Take a bowl and combine the egg, ricotta, 75g Parmesan and parsley, until smooth
6. Remove the parchment from the aubergine and wipe off the salt
7. Take a tablespoon of the ricotta mixture and place on top of each round of aubergine, spreading with a knife
8. Place in the freezer for a while to set
9. Take a bowl and add the two eggs, the pork rinds, parmesan and seasonings, and combine
10. Remove the aubergine from the freezer and coat each one in the mixture completely
11. Place back in the freezer for 45 minutes
12. Cook in the air fryer for 8 minutes at 250ºC

Zingy Roasted Carrots

Servings: 4
Cooking Time:xx

Ingredients:

- 500g carrots
- 1 tsp olive oil
- 1 tsp cayenne pepper
- Salt and pepper for seasoning

Directions:

1. Peel the carrots and cut them into chunks, around 2" in size
2. Preheat your air fryer to 220ºC
3. Add the carrots to a bowl with the olive oil and cayenne and toss to coat
4. Place in the fryer and cook for 15 minutes, giving them a stir halfway through
5. Season before serving

Shishito Peppers

Servings: 2
Cooking Time:xx

Ingredients:

- 200g shishito peppers
- Salt and pepper to taste
- ½ tbsp avocado oil
- 75g grated cheese
- 2 limes

Directions:

1. Rinse the peppers
2. Place in a bowl and mix with oil, salt and pepper
3. Place in the air fryer and cook at 175ºC for 10 minutes
4. Place on a serving plate and sprinkle with cheese

Butternut Squash Fries

Servings: 4
Cooking Time:xx

Ingredients:

- 400g butternut squash, cut into sticks
- 1 tbsp olive oil
- 2 tbsp bagel seasoning
- 1 tsp fresh chopped rosemary

Directions:

1. Preheat air fryer to 200ºC
2. Drizzle butternut squash with olive oil mix to coat
3. Add to the air fryer, cook for about 22 minutes until golden brown, stirring every 4 minutes
4. Sprinkle with bagel seasoning to serve

Desserts Recipes

Banana And Nutella Sandwich

Servings: 2
Cooking Time:xx

Ingredients:

- Softened butter
- 4 slices white bread
- 25g chocolate spread
- 1 banana

Directions:

1. Preheat the air fryer to 185ºC
2. Spread butter on one side of all the bread slices
3. Spread chocolate spread on the other side of each slice
4. Add sliced banana to two slices of bread then add the other slice of bread to each
5. Cut in half diagonally to form triangles
6. Place in the air fryer and cook for 5 minutes turn over and cook for another 2 minutes

Cinnamon-maple Pineapple Kebabs

Servings: 2
Cooking Time:xx

Ingredients:

- 4 x pineapple strips, roughly 2 x 2 cm/¾ x ¾ in. by length of pineapple
- 1 teaspoon maple syrup
- ½ teaspoon vanilla extract
- ¼ teaspoon ground cinnamon
- Greek or plant-based yogurt and grated lime zest, to serve

Directions:

1. Line the air-fryer with an air-fryer liner or a piece of pierced parchment paper. Preheat the air-fryer to 180ºC/350ºF.
2. Stick small metal skewers through the pineapple lengthways. Mix the maple syrup and vanilla extract together, then drizzle over the pineapple and sprinkle over the cinnamon.
3. Add the skewers to the preheated lined air-fryer and air-fry for 15 minutes, turning once. If there is any maple-vanilla mixture left after the initial drizzle, then drizzle this over the pineapple during cooking too. Serve with yogurt and lime zest.

Apple Pie

Servings: 2
Cooking Time:xx

Ingredients:

- 1 packet of ready made pastry
- 1 apple, chopped
- 2 tsp lemon juice
- 1 tsp cinnamon
- 2 tbsp sugar
- ½ tsp vanilla extract
- 1 tbsp butter
- 1 beaten egg
- 1 tbsp raw sugar

Directions:

1. Preheat the air fryer to 160ºC
2. Line a baking tin with pastry
3. Mix the apple, lemon juice, cinnamon, sugar and vanilla in a bowl
4. Pour the apple mix into the tin with the pastry, top with chunks of butter
5. Cover with a second piece of pastry, place three slits in the top of the pastry
6. Brush the pastry with beaten egg and sprinkle with raw sugar
7. Place in the air fryer and cook for 30 minutes

Chocolate Dipped Biscuits

Servings: 6
Cooking Time:xx

Ingredients:

- 225g self raising flour
- 100g sugar
- 100g butter
- 50g milk chocolate
- 1 egg beaten
- 1 tsp vanilla essence

Directions:

1. Add the flour, butter and sugar to a bowl and rub together
2. Add the egg and vanilla, mix to form a dough
3. Split the dough into 6 and form into balls
4. Place in the air fryer cook at 180ºC for 15 minutes
5. Melt the chocolate, dip the cooked biscuits into the chocolate and half cover

Cinnamon Bites

Servings: 8
Cooking Time:xx

Ingredients:

- 200g flour
- 200g whole wheat flour
- 2 tbsp sugar
- 1 tsp baking powder
- ¼ tsp cinnamon
- 3 tbsp water
- ¼ tsp salt
- 4 tbsp butter
- 25ml milk
- Cooking spray
- 350g powdered sugar

Directions:

1. Mix together flour, sugar, baking powder and salt in a bowl
2. Add the butter and mix well
3. Add the milk and mix to form a dough
4. Knead until dough is smooth, cut into 16 pieces
5. Roll each piece into a small ball
6. Coat the air fryer with cooking spray and heat to 175ºC
7. Add the balls to the air fryer and cook for 12 minutes
8. Mix the powdered sugar and water together, decorate

Profiteroles

Servings: 9
Cooking Time:xx
Ingredients:

- 100g butter
- 200g plain flour
- 6 eggs
- 300ml water
- 2 tsp vanilla extract
- 300ml whipped cream
- 100g milk chocolate
- 2 tbsp whipped cream
- 50g butter
- 2 tsp icing sugar

Directions:

1. Preheat the air fryer to 170°C
2. Place the butter and water in a pan over a medium heat, bring to the boil, remove from the heat and stir in the flour
3. Return to the heat stirring until a dough is formed
4. Mix in the eggs and stir until mixture is smooth, make into profiterole shapes and cook in the air fryer for 10 minutes
5. For the filling whisk together 300ml whipped cream, vanilla extract and the icing sugar
6. For the topping place the butter, 2tbsp whipped cream and chocolate in a bowl and melt over a pan of hot water until mixed together
7. Pipe the filling into the roles and finish off with a chocolate topping

Birthday Cheesecake

Servings: 8
Cooking Time:xx
Ingredients:

- 6 Digestive biscuits
- 50g melted butter
- 800g soft cheese
- 500g caster sugar
- 4 tbsp cocoa powder
- 6 eggs
- 2 tbsp honey
- 1 tbsp vanilla

Directions:

1. Flour a spring form tin to prevent sticking
2. Crush the biscuits and then mix with the melted butter, press into the bottom and sides of the tin
3. Mix the caster sugar and soft cheese with an electric mixer. Add 5 eggs, honey and vanilla. Mix well
4. Spoon half the mix into the pan and pat down well. Place in the air fryer and cook at 180°C for 20 minutes then 160°C for 15 minutes and then 150°C for 20 minutes
5. Mix the cocoa and the last egg into the remaining mix. Spoon over the over the bottom layer and place in the fridge. Chill for 11 hours

Mini Egg Buns

Servings: 8
Cooking Time:xx

Ingredients:

- 100g self raising flour
- 100g caster sugar
- 100g butter
- 2 eggs
- 2 tbsp honey
- 1 tbsp vanilla essence
- 300g soft cheese
- 100g icing sugar
- 2 packets of Mini Eggs

Directions:

1. Cream the butter and sugar together until light and fluffy, beat in the eggs one at a time
2. Add the honey and vanilla essence, fold in the flour a bit at a time
3. Divide the mix into 8 bun cases and place in the air fryer. Cook at 180ºC for about 20 minutes
4. Cream the soft cheese and icing sugar together to make the topping
5. Allow the buns to cool, pipe on the topping mix and add mini eggs

Peanut Butter & Chocolate Baked Oats

Servings:9
Cooking Time:xx

Ingredients:

- 150 g/1 heaped cup rolled oats/quick-cooking oats
- 50 g/⅓ cup dark chocolate chips or buttons
- 300 ml/1¼ cups milk or plant-based milk
- 50 g/3½ tablespoons Greek or plant-based yogurt
- 1 tablespoon runny honey or maple syrup
- ½ teaspoon ground cinnamon or ground ginger
- 65 g/scant ⅓ cup smooth peanut butter

Directions:

1. Stir all the ingredients together in a bowl, then transfer to a baking dish that fits your air-fryer drawer.
2. Preheat the air-fryer to 180ºC/350ºF.
3. Add the baking dish to the preheated air-fryer and air-fry for 10 minutes. Remove from the air-fryer and serve hot, cut into 9 squares.

Fruit Crumble

Servings: 2
Cooking Time:xx

Ingredients:

- 1 diced apple
- 75g frozen blackberries
- 25g brown rice flour
- 2 tbsp sugar
- ½ tsp cinnamon
- 2 tbsp butter

Directions:

1. Preheat air fryer to 150ºC
2. Mix apple and blackberries in an air fryer safe baking pan
3. In a bowl mix the flour, sugar, cinnamon and butter, spoon over the fruit
4. Cook for 15 minutes

Chocolate And Berry Pop Tarts

Servings:8
Cooking Time:10 Minutes
Ingredients:

- For the filling:
- 50 g / 1.8 oz fresh raspberries
- 50 g / 1.8 oz fresh strawberries
- 100 g / 3.5 oz granulated sugar
- 1 tsp corn starch
- For the pastry:
- 1 sheet puff pastry
- For the frosting:
- 4 tbsp powdered sugar
- 2 tbsp maple syrup or honey
- Chocolate sprinkles

Directions:

1. Preheat the air fryer to 180 °C / 350 °F and line the mesh basket with parchment paper or grease it with olive oil.
2. Make the filling by combining the strawberries, raspberries, and granulated sugar in a saucepan. Place on medium heat until the mixture starts to boil. When it begins to boil, turn the temperature down to a low setting. Use a spoon to break up the berries and forms a smooth mixture.
3. Stir in the corn starch and let the mixture simmer for 1-2 minutes. Remove the saucepan from the heat and set aside to cool while you prepare the pastry.
4. Roll out the large sheet of puff pastry and cut it into 8 equal rectangles.
5. Spoon 2 tbsp of the cooled berry filling onto one side of each rectangle. Fold over the other side of each puff pastry rectangle to cover the filling. Press the sides down with a fork or using your fingers to seal the filling into the pastry.
6. Transfer the puff pastry rectangles into the lined air fryer basket. Cook for 10-12 minutes until the pastry is golden and crispy.
7. Meanwhile, make the frosting. Whisk together the powdered sugar, maple syrup or honey, and chocolate chips in a bowl until well combined.
8. Carefully spread a thin layer of frosting in the centre of each pop tart. Allow the frosting to set before serving.

Apple And Cinnamon Empanadas

Servings: 12
Cooking Time:xx
Ingredients:

- 12 empanada wraps
- 2 diced apples
- 2 tbsp honey
- 1 tsp vanilla extract
- 1 tsp cinnamon
- ⅛ tsp nutmeg
- Olive oil spray
- 2 tsp cornstarch
- 1 tsp water

Directions:

1. Place apples, cinnamon, honey, vanilla and nutmeg in a pan cook for 2-3 minutes until apples are soft
2. Mix the cornstarch and water add to the pan and cook for 30 seconds
3. Add the apple mix to each of the empanada wraps
4. Roll the wrap in half, pinch along the edges, fold the edges in then continue to roll to seal
5. Place in the air fryer and cook at 200ºC for 8 minutes, turn and cook for another 10 minutes

Lemon Buns

Servings: 12
Cooking Time:xx

Ingredients:

- 100g butter
- 100g caster sugar
- 2 eggs
- 100g self raising flour
- ½ tsp vanilla essence
- 1 tsp cherries
- 50g butter
- 100g icing sugar
- ½ small lemon rind and juice

Directions:

1. Preheat the air fryer to 170°C
2. Cream the 100g butter, sugar and vanilla together until light and fluffy
3. Beat in the eggs one at a time adding a little flour with each
4. Fold in the remaining flour
5. Half fill bun cases with the mix, place in the air fryer and cook for 8 minutes
6. Cream 50g butter then mix in the icing sugar, stir in the lemon
7. Slice the top off each bun and create a butterfly shape using the icing to hold together. Add a 1/3 cherry to each one

Pop Tarts

Servings: 6
Cooking Time:xx

Ingredients:

- 200g strawberries quartered
- 25g sugar
- ½ pack ready made pie crust
- Cooking spray
- 50g powdered sugar
- 1 ½ tsp lemon juice
- 1 tbsp sprinkles

Directions:

1. Stir together strawberries and sugar in a bowl
2. Allow to stand for 15 minutes then microwave on high for 10 minutes stirring halfway through
3. Roll out pie crust int0 12 inch circle, cut into 12 rectangles
4. Spoon mix onto 6 of the rectangles
5. Brush the edges with water and top with the remaining rectangles
6. Press around the edges with a fork to seal
7. Place in the air fryer and cook at 175°C for about 10 minutes
8. Mix together powdered sugar and decorate add sprinkles

Cherry Pies

Servings: 6
Cooking Time:xx

Ingredients:

- 300g prepared shortcrust pastry
- 75g cherry pie filling
- Cooking spray
- 3 tbsp icing sugar
- ½ tsp milk

Directions:

1. Cut out 6 pies with a cookie cutter
2. Add 1 ½ tbsp filling to each pie
3. Fold the dough in half and seal around the edges with a fork
4. Place in the air fryer, spray with cooking spray
5. Cook at 175ºC for 10 minutes
6. Mix icing sugar and milk and drizzled over cooled pies to serve

French Toast Sticks

Servings: 12
Cooking Time:xx

Ingredients:

- 2 eggs
- 25g milk
- 1 tbsp melted butter
- 1 tsp vanilla extract
- 1 tsp cinnamon
- 4 slices bread, cut into thirds
- 1 tsp icing sugar

Directions:

1. Mix eggs, milk, butter, vanilla and cinnamon together in a bowl
2. Line the air fryer with parchment paper
3. Dip each piece of bread into the egg mixture
4. Place in the air fryer and cook at 190ºC for 6 minutes, turn over and cook for another 3 minutes
5. Sprinkle with icing sugar to serve

Melting Moments

Servings: 9
Cooking Time:xx

Ingredients:

- 100g butter
- 75g caster sugar
- 150g self raising flour
- 1 egg
- 50g white chocolate
- 3 tbsp desiccated coconut
- 1 tsp vanilla essence

Directions:

1. Preheat the air fryer to 180°C
2. Cream together the butter and sugar, beat in the egg and vanilla
3. Bash the white chocolate into small pieces
4. Add the flour and chocolate and mix well
5. Roll into 9 small balls and cover in coconut
6. Place in the air fryer and cook for 8 minutes and a further 6 minutes at 160°C

White Chocolate And Raspberry Loaf

Servings:8
Cooking Time:1 Hour 10 Minutes

Ingredients:

- 400 g / 14 oz plain flour
- 2 tsp baking powder
- 1 tsp ground cinnamon
- ½ tsp salt
- 3 eggs, beaten
- 50 g / 3.5 oz granulated sugar
- 50 g / 3.5 oz brown sugar
- 100 g / 3.5 oz white chocolate chips
- 100 g / 3.5 oz fresh raspberries
- 1 tbsp cocoa powder
- 4 tbsp milk
- 1 tsp vanilla extract

Directions:

1. Preheat the air fryer to 150 °C / 300 °F and line a loaf tin with parchment paper.
2. Combine the plain flour, baking powder, ground cinnamon, and salt in a large mixing bowl.
3. Whisk eggs into the bowl, then stir in the granulated sugar and brown sugar. Mix well before folding in the white chocolate chips, fresh raspberries, cocoa powder, milk, and vanilla extract.
4. Stir the mixture until it is lump-free and transfer into a lined loaf tin. Place the loaf tin into the lined air fryer basket, close the lid, and cook for 30-40 minutes.
5. The cake should be golden and set by the end of the cooking process. Insert a knife into the centre of the cake. It should come out dry when the cake is fully cooked.
6. Remove the cake from the air fryer, still in the loaf tin. Set aside to cool on a drying rack for 20-30 minutes before cutting into slices and serving.

Breakfast Muffins

Servings:4
Cooking Time:xx
Ingredients:

- 1 eating apple, cored and grated
- 40 g/2 heaped tablespoons maple syrup
- 40 ml/3 tablespoons oil (avocado, olive or coconut), plus extra for greasing
- 1 egg
- 40 ml/3 tablespoons milk (plant-based if you wish)
- 90 g/scant ¾ cup brown rice flour
- 50 g/½ cup ground almonds
- ¾ teaspoon ground cinnamon
- ⅛ teaspoon ground cloves
- ¼ teaspoon salt
- 1 teaspoon baking powder
- Greek or plant-based yogurt and fresh fruit, to serve

Directions:

1. In a bowl mix the grated apple, maple syrup, oil, egg and milk. In another bowl mix the rice flour, ground almonds, cinnamon, cloves, salt and baking powder. Combine the wet ingredients with the dry, mixing until there are no visible patches of the flour mixture left. Grease 4 ramekins and divide the batter equally between them.
2. Preheat the air-fryer to 160°C/325°F.
3. Add the ramekins to the preheated air-fryer and air-fry for 12 minutes. Check the muffins are cooked by inserting a cocktail stick/toothpick into the middle of one of the muffins. If it comes out clean, the muffins are ready; if not, cook for a further couple of minutes.
4. Allow to cool in the ramekins, then remove and serve with your choice of yogurt and fresh fruit.

Shortbread Cookies

Servings: 2
Cooking Time:xx
Ingredients:

- 250g flour
- 75g sugar
- 175g butter
- 1 tbsp vanilla essence
- Chocolate buttons for decoration

Directions:

1. Preheat air fryer to 180°C
2. Place all ingredients apart from the chocolate into a bowl and rub together
3. Form into dough and roll out. Cut into heart shapes using a cookie cutter
4. Place in the air fryer and cook for 10 minutes
5. Place the chocolate buttons onto the shortbread and cook for another 10 minutes at 160°C

Appendix : Recipes Index

A

B

C

E

F

G

H

Q

R

S

T

V

W

Z

Printed in Great Britain
by Amazon

26787904R00051